Probiotics in Improving Human Health

About the Author

Dr. Renu Agrawal is Ex. Chief Scientist, CSIR-CFTRI and Rural Development Programme Coordinator, Mysore. She is a science columnist, reviewer, science reformer, counsellor, author of books and works for social upliftment. She has represented India as a team leader taking scientific delegation for Asia meet at Indonesia, Bali nominated by DST, Government of India. She had her PhD from University of Rajasthan, Jaipur. Her areas of specialization include biotransformation and probiotics. She has received many externally funded project grants as principal investigator from DBT (Department of Biotechnology) and DST (Department of Science and Technology) Govt. of India and Bilateral International programmes with Bulgaria and Argentina. Her path breaking and innovative research is evidenced by her publications. She has developed many innovative functional foods and technologies oriented towards improving health by natural means. She has guided students for M.Sc, M. phil and PhD in Biotechnology and Microbiology. She has published more than 60 research papers in peer reviewed national and international journals. She has presented more than 160 papers in various national and international conferences and delivered more than 300 talks. She has 20 patents to her credit.

She has been honored as **Fellows** of "Fellow of Association of Microbiologists of India", Fellow member of International Society of Biotechnology', Fellow of National Academy of Biological Sciences and "Fellow Society of Applied Biotechnology".

She is a reviewer of many national and international journals. She has authored a book on Probiotics and many book chapters including from Marcell Dekkar, USA and Taylor and Francis, UK. Her work has won many best paper awards at the national and international conferences. She has taught as faculty of M.Sc Food Technology at CFTRI and to ACSIR students. She has served as the president of 'Association of Microbiologists of India", Mysore chapter and has been a member of many international Technical Advisory Boards.

She has been nominated to Co-Chair the Expert Committees on Scheme for Young Scientists and Technologists (SYST), Department of Science and Technology, Govt. of India.

After retirement she is working as a project advisor (CFTRI).

Probiotics in Improving Human Health

Renu Agrawal
FAMI, FNABS, FSAB, FISBT
Chief Scientist
Food Microbiology
Central Food Technological Research Institute, Mysore

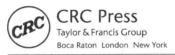

CRC Press
Taylor & Francis Group
Boca Raton London New York

CRC Press is an imprint of the
Taylor & Francis Group, an **informa** business

NEW INDIA PUBLISHING AGENCY
New Delhi – 110 034

CRC Press
Taylor & Francis Group
6000 Broken Sound Parkway NW, Suite 300
Boca Raton, FL 33487-2742

© 2020 by New India Publishing Agency

CRC Press is an imprint of the Taylor & Francis Group, an informa business

No claim to original U.S. Government works

International Standard Book Number-13: 978-0-367-49267-0 (Hardback)

This book contains information obtained from authentic and highly regarded sources. Reasonable efforts have been made to publish reliable data and information, but the author and publisher cannot assume responsibility for the validity of all materials or the consequences of their use. The authors and publishers have attempted to trace the copyright holders of all material reproduced in this publication and apologize to copyright holders if permission to publish in this form has not been obtained. If any copyright material has not been acknowledged please write and let us know so we may rectify in any future reprint.

Except as permitted under U.S. Copyright Law, no part of this book may be reprinted, reproduced, transmitted, or utilized in any form by any electronic, mechanical, or other means, now known or hereafter invented, including photocopying, microfilming, and recording, or in any information storage or retrieval system, without written permission from the publishers.

For permission to photocopy or use material electronically from this work, please access www.copyright.com (http://www.copyright.com/) or contact the Copyright Clearance Center, Inc. (CCC), 222 Rosewood Drive, Danvers, MA 01923, 978-750-8400. CCC is a not-for-profit organization that provides licenses and registration for a variety of users. For organizations that have been granted a photocopy license by the CCC, a separate system of payment has been arranged.

Trademark notice: Product or corporate names may be trademarks or registered trademarks, and are used only for identification and explanation without intent to infringe.

Print edition not for sale in South Asia (India, Sri Lanka, Nepal, Bangladesh, Pakistan or Bhutan)

Library of Congress Cataloging-in-Publication Data
A catalog record has been requested

Visit the Taylor & Francis Web site at
http://www.taylorandfrancis.com

and the CRC Press Web site at
http://www.crcpress.com

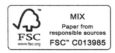

Printed in the United Kingdom
by Henry Ling Limited

World Noni Research Foundation
12, Rajiv Gandhi Road Perungudi, Chennai – 600 096, India
Phone: 044-49011111; Fax: 044-49011115, E-mail: kvptr@yahoo.com

Dr. K. V. Peter, Ph.D. FNASc., FNAAS., FNABS, FHSI
FISVS, FFSGP
Former Vice-Chancellor, KAU
Director, World Noni Research Foundation
No. 12, Srinivasa Nagar, 2nd Street
Rajiv Gandhi Road, Old Mahabalipuram Road
Perungudi, Chennai – 600 096

Chennai - 600096
24, June 2016

FOREWORD

The book "Probiotics in Improving Human Health" authored by Dr. Renu Agrawal aims at creating awareness about probiotics and their importance in leading a healthy balanced life. Probiotic have made a special place in human nutrition and therapy as they are natural and fall under the GRAS category. There is something novel and new happening in this area of research everyday, so that there is a need to have all the data compiled and updated from time to time to help the researchers and the population at large.

A century of research in this area resulted in several probiotic products which are now available in the market. This book aims at enlisting the various developments which have taken place in the field starting from isolation of microbes to the health implication which probiotics can bring about.

Today a number of products have come into the market. The medical practitioners are also recommending probiotic in different forms to the patients especially affected by new life style diseases obesity, diabetes, cardiovascular diseases and overweight. In fact the scientists are working on probiotics since a century. Today, it has come a long way with the recent developments in formulation manufacture, packing, storage and marketing.

Chapter 1, deals with the Introduction to probiotics. Chapter 2, deals with the probiotic Properties, Selection and Benefits. Chapter 3, deals with the classification of probiotics, Chapter 4, deals with the diseases known to be improved by probiotics. The therapeutic roles of probiotics for improving the gut-health have been brought out with recent research work. This section covers the Intestinal disorders, their influence of resident intestinal micro flora on the development and function and also peptides and immuno-modulation. The sub section covers diseases like Diarrhoea. *Helxobxur priori* infection, Tumor, Bowel, HIV, lactase deficiency and IIID. The other sub section deals with Non-intestinal disorders like Allergy, immunity, urinary tract infection, bacterial vaginosis, Arthritis, mineral absorption. carcinogenesis, hypercholesterolemia, denial caries. Tract infection, hypertension, kidney stone, surgical wound infections, chronic fatigue syndrome and lowering blood pressure.

Improvement of probiotic strains can give better functional results strain improvement for better results is discussed in the next section. There are only limited information about the mechanism of action of probiotics. A section separately covers the Mechanism of action followed by Innovative new Probiotic products. While it is good to have new products, getting them to the market is a challenge. Industries are keen to know about the business with probiotic products. A section have been allocated to deal with the *pros* and *cons* of the Probiotic Business Environment. With numerous probiotic products in the global market, consumers are seldom convinced about the reliability of these products. One section of this book focuses on the functional foods and reliability and development of probiotic dosage forms. This is followed by the efficacy of probiotics. Preservation of probiotics by freeze drying and microencapsulation techniques for shelf life extension are also covered. No product can be utilized by the human beings unless clinical trials are conducted and therefore the author has written a separate section on Animal and Clinical studies conducted on probiotics / probiotic products. For any product to be kept safe for a longer time it is important to have a good packaging. The book has been unique in presenting a dedicated section on the role of packaging to enhance shelf life of probiotic products followed by Multifunctional genetically improved probiotic and biomedical trend in the 21st century. The author has dealt with the Market Trend around the world, what new researches are needed, what trials are needed and how the consumers and industry can benefit and what will be the future implications of probiotics. *Saccharomyces* spp. is a fast developing probiotic and therefore a section has been written on the yeast cells. Looking into the criticality on the safety of the culture a section has been written on the Safety of probiotic culture.

This book provides a very comprehensive review starting from the fundamentals of probiotic organisms to their therapeutic and industrial aspects and efficacy as adjudged by clinical trials. It provides the most recent updates in this area with a holistic approach.

The author has been working in the field of probiotic for more than two decades and has remarkable experience in the field of probiotic organisms. I am sure that this book will be very useful not only for academicians and students, but also for industries preparing probiotics products. The book will be of great use to the food scientists and technologists and I recommend that targeted readers especially food technologists read and benefit immensely from this book. I appreciate Dr Renu Agrawal a Fellow of National Academy of Biological Sciences, Chennai for the time, effort and patience taken. I congratulate, New India Publishing Agency New Delhi (www.nipabooks.com) for publishing the book.

K.V. Peter

PREFACE

Today the population is concerned about many side effects of antibiotics like inflammation which is happening due to decrease in immunity and all this is causing a lot of diseases. Foremost thing for good health, is to have a healthy gut which can happen only when it has higher number of—good bacteria over pathogens in the gut.

Today, in the 21st century the natural means of improving gut bacteria are taking a top position and that is the use of probiotics. These are helpful in digestion, in improving urogenital diseases, cancer, cardiovascular and many allergies.

This book has attempted to bring an insight from isolation, characterization, properties, inhibition of various diseases, shelf stability and market potential of probiotics, validation in animals and human clinical trials.

Probiotic foods which are dairy or non-dairy provide healthful attributes. Therefore, these foods are a part of the book.

Author

CONTENTS

Foreword v

Preface vii

1. Introduction 1
2. Probiotic Properties: Selection and Benefits 7
3. Classification of Probiotics 17
4. Diseases Known to be Inhibited by Probiotics 19
5. Mechanism of Action of Lactic Acid Bacteria 67
6. Innovative New Probiotic Products 71
7. Animal and Clinical Studies 99
8. Role of Packaging to Enhance Shelf Life of Probiotic Products ... 103
9. Market Trend on Probiotic Around the World 115
10. Future Implications of Probiotics 117
11. *Saccharomyces* spp. As Probiotics 121

References 127

1
INTRODUCTION

Newer technologies involve fermentation by specific strains of lactic acid bacteria which bring specific fermentation under controlled conditions to a specific fermented product with enhanced organoleptic, nutritional and therapeutic qualities. Today health is of primary concern. It is important to have nutritionally balanced food with good bacteria. For this, probiotic foods top the list. The functional food concept was initially developed in Japan in 1990's as there were many side effects of allopathic medicines. A regulatory system has been initiated by the ministry of health and welfare to approve certain foods to improve health. These are now recognized as Foods for specialized health use (FOSHU). According to American dietic association (ADA) these foods are potential healthful food or food ingredients that may provide health benefits beyond the traditional nutrients. Probiotics are beneficial microorganisms. Probiotic foods as yogurt and sauerkraut are very well known. Fermentation increases the nutrient content and taste with the shelf life. They also support the immune system. There is a lot of development in functional foods, organic foods and national foods around the world. The global demand is increasing by 15-20% every year. Caplice and Fitzgerald (1999) have studied the role of microorganisms in food production and preservation. Carr *et al.* (2002) have done a good survey on lactic acid bacteria.

Lactic acid bacteria are non-spore forming, gram positive and catalase negative without cytochromes, non-aerobic or aerotolerant, fastidious, acid-tolerant and strictly fermentative bacteria with lactic acid as the major end product during sugar fermentation. Lactic acid bacteria are safe, non toxic, non pathogenic and non-spore forming. Vanaja *et al.* (2011) have studied the differences in biochemical and electrophoretic properties in native *Lactobacillus plantarum* and probiotic culture strain *Lactobacillus plantarum* cfr on adaptation to GIT conditions with functional properties. Viable LAB of human origin helps to restore normal intestinal microbial functions, alleviating disease symptoms in patients with GIT infection, stimulating the immune system, exposing anti cancerous and anti atherosclerosis effects (Lin and Chang, 2000; McFarland, 2000; Isolauri *et al.*, 2001). Vanitha and Agrawal (2012) purified a protein from probiotic *Leuconostoc mesenteroides* active against *V. cholerae*. The antioxidative effect of LAB has been reported only recently (Kaizu *et al.*, 1993; Lin and Yen, 1999; Lin and Chang, 2000; Kullisaar *et al.*, 2002). A wide variety of reactive oxygen species are continuously produced in the human body (de Zwart *et al.*, 1999; Juránek and Bezek, 2005). Damage caused by reactive oxygen species plays a substantial role in the pathogenesis of human diseases such as cancer, cardiovascular diseases, allergies and atherosclerosis (Agerholm *et al.*, 2000). Bultman (2014) have shown that microbiome plays a vital role in cancer Carcinogenesis. There is not much data about the antioxidative ability of LAB available. LAB genera have been isolated from various fermented foods namely *Lactobacillus, Pediococcus, Enterococcus, Lactococcus, Leuconostoc, Oenococcus, Streptococcus, Tetrazenococcus, Carnobacterium, Vagococcus* and *Weissella* (Stiles and Holzapfel, 1997; Carr *et al.*, 2002; Salminen *et al.*, 2003). Erdogrul and Erbilir (2006) have isolated and characterized *Lactobacillus bulgaricus* and *Lactobacillus casei* from various foods. Charteris *et al.* (1997) have done a selective detection, enumeration and identification of potentially probiotic *Lactobacillus* and *Bifidobacterium* species in mixed bacterial populations. LAB produces organic acids during fermentation which is mostly lactic acid and is the characteristic fermentative product. This reduces the pH of the substrate to a level where the growth of pathogenic, putrefactive, and toxinogenic bacteria are inhibited (Holzapfel *et al.*, 2001). LAB has been given GRAS (generally recognized as safe) status in foods (Donohue and Salminen, 1996). Satokari *et al.* (2003) have looked into the molecular approaches for the detection and identification of *Bifidobacteria* and *Lactobacilli* in the human gastrointestinal tract. Many species of LAB can also act as biopreservers and some of them are exploited commercially. Wang *et al.* (2006) have studied commensal microbes as a potentially important avenue in transmitting antibiotic resistance genes. Phenotypic identification of LAB in dairy products is mainly done morphologically, physiologically and biochemically being indispensable tools (Badis *et al.*, 2004). Badis *et al.* (2004) have identified and studied the technological properties of lactic acid bacteria isolated from raw goat milk of four Algerian races.

Fermented foods have beneficial bacteria which keep the digestive tract healthy and protect them against virulent pathogens that cause food borne illnesses. Use of antibiotics kills the beneficial microorganisms along with the pathogens. Probiotic foods can prevent or alleviate many health disorders ranging from allergy and asthma to yeast infection and heart diseases that result from food borne infections and antibiotic resistance. Probiotic foods provide special nutritional and therapeutic properties over the traditional ones. For commercialization extreme modifications are to be done. There are fermented foods based on vegetables, beans, and cereal grains. Fermented foods are nutritious and easily fit into the daily diet. These are carriers of health promoting microbes that reach the intestine when consumed (Anonymous, 2010). Williams *et al.* (2006) have discussed functional foods as great opportunity for developing countries.

A large population of live bacterial cells (10^{14}) colonizes in the human GI tract which may change depending on the physiology of the host and bacterial interaction.

The microbial flora influences the functioning of the gut associated lymphoid tissue (GALT). At the time of birth the baby's intestine is sterile but within 48 h almost 10^9/g bacteria are found in the feces (Hudault, 1994). Facultative anaerobic bacteria like *E.coli* and *Streptococcus* colonize. After 2 to 4 d other bacteria like *Bifidobacterium, Bacteroides* and *Clostridium* also inhabit the intestine. The flora may be different in the breast fed and bottle fed babies. Bacteria like *Bifidobacterium, E.coli* and *Streptococcus* are found in breast fed infants whereas when bottle fed *Bacteroides, Clostridia* and *Enterobacteria* are also found. Goldin *et al.* (1980) have shown the effect of diet on *Lactobacillus acidophilus*.

1. Probiotics in Health

Probiotic bacteria provide specific health benefits when consumed as a food component (Gaurner and Malagelada, 2003). There are lots of studies on the health benefits of probiotic fermented foods (Dugas *et al.*, 1999; Scherezenmeir and de Vrese, 2001; Dunne *et al.*, 2001). Eighty species of *Lactobacilli* have been recognized and characterized (Satokari *et al.*, 2003). Some of the proposed health benefits provided by probiotic species include reduction of diarrhea (Yan and Polk, 2006), prevention of colon cancer, lowering of cholesterol and enhancement of the immune system (Piaia *et al.*, 2003; Jones, 2002; Tavan *et al.*, 2002). These organisms are strictly fermentative which could be aero tolerant or anaerobic and have a complex nutritional requirement. These are widely present in nature and are naturally present in raw milk. These Gram-positive bacteria play an important role in many foods and feed fermentations. These include representatives of the genus *Lactobacillus, Lactococcus, Pediococcus* and *Leuconostoc* (Guessas and Kihal, 2004). Goldin *et al.* (1987) have shown reduction in cell number of *Clostridium difficile* with probiotics. Goldin and Gorbach (1992) have written a comprehensive article on probiotics in relation to humans.

These are known to produce volatile compounds which produce flavors. Ha *et al.* (1987) investigated the effect of cellular membrane with different fatty acid composition on the growth of *Lactobacillus delbrueckii*. Corsetti *et al.* (1998) reported the production of caprylic acid from *L. sanfranciscensis* which is isolated from sourdough and plays a key role for inhibitory activity against bacteria and moulds. Conjugated linoleic acid (CLA) has gained considerable importance because of its potentially beneficial biological effects. Composition of CLA inhibits the initiation of carcinogenesis (Hayatsu *et al.*, 1981). Kankaanpaa *et al.* (2004) reported that whether the free linoleic acid, γ - linolenicacid, arachidonic acid, α-linolenic acid or docosahexaenoic acid in the growth medium alters the fatty acid composition of *Lactobacilli*.

The main uses are:

- Prevention of gastrointestinal problems
- Improving immune system
- Reduction of cholesterol
- Lowering of blood pressure
- Reduction of allergic symptoms
- Suppression of pathogenic microorganisms (antimicrobial effect)
- Prevention of osteoporosis
- Prevention of urogenital infections

Definition of probiotics

The word "probiotic" comes from Greek language pro-bios which means for life. The use of lactic acid bacteria as feed supplements goes back to pre-Christian times when fermented milks were consumed by humans. It was not until the beginning of this century that Metchnikoff, working at the Pasteur Institute in Parishad put a scientific basis. In 1908, he proposed the beneficial effects of probiotic microorganisms on human health. Metchnikoff hypothesized that the health of Bulgarians and long life was because of the consumption of fermented milk products containing *Lactobacillus* spp. These bacteria affect the gut microflora positively and decrease the microbial toxic activity (Gismondo *et al.*, 1999; Chuayana *et al.*, 2003). The term probiotic was used in 1965 for the first time by Lilley and Stillwell to describe substances which stimulate the growth of other microorganisms. The word probiotic was used based on its mechanism and the effect on human health. According to Parker (1974) these organisms contributed to the intestinal microbial biota. Fuller (1989) defined probiotic as a live microbial supplement which affects host's health positively by improving its intestinal microbial balance. Guarino *et al.* (1997) defined probiotics as —"living microorganisms, which exert health benefits upon ingestion in certain numbers beyond inherent basic nutrition". According to many other scientists probiotics were defined as:

Salminen *et al.* (1998) "A live microbial food ingredient that is beneficial to health".

Naidu *et al.* (1999) "A microbial dietary adjuvant that beneficially affects the host physiology by modulating mucosal and systemic immunity, as well as improving nutritional and microbial balance in the intestinal tract".

Schrezenmeir and de Vrese (2001) "A preparation of a product containing viable, defined microorganisms in sufficient numbers, which alter the microflora in the host and exert beneficial health effects".

FAO/WHO (2002a) "Live microorganisms which when administered in adequate amounts confer health benefit on the host".

Probiotics are used in a large variety of fields relevant to human and animal health. Probiotic products contain one or several species of probiotic bacteria. Most of the products are dairy based like fermented milk or as lyophilized powders in the form of tablets. The oral consumption of probiotic microorganisms produces a protective effect on the gut flora. Many studies suggest that probiotics have beneficial effects on microbial disorders of the gut. They are known to have a positive therapeutic effect against traveller's diarrhoea, antibiotic associated diarrhoea and acute diarrhoea (Gismondo *et al.*, 1999; Ouwehand *et al.*, 1999a). In the human intestinal tract more than 400 bacterial species exist. A number of factors may change the balance from potentially beneficial or health promoting bacteria like *Lactobacilli* and *Bifidobacteria* to potentially harmful or pathogenic microorganisms like *Clostridia* species that makes the host more susceptible to illnesses. In this case the prevalence of the beneficial bacteria must be supported (Shoria and Ahmad, 2015). Use of probiotics helps to protect the host from various intestinal disorders by increasing the number of beneficial bacteria (Fooks *et al.*, 1999). The most commonly used microorganisms in probiotic products are the lactic acid bacteria (LAB) and it is important to know how these LAB affect the immune status of the consumer. The probiotic approach is attractive because it is a reconstitution of the natural condition which means repairing a deficiency rather than the addition of foreign chemicals like antibiotics to the body which may have toxic consequences or, as in the case of antibiotics induce resístance and compromise subsequent therapy. The discovery that probiotics can stimulate an immune response (Fuller and Perdigon *et al.*, 2000) provides a scientific basis for some of the observed probiotic effects. The probiotics which are used to feed both man and animals are given in Table (1).

Table 1: Microorganisms used in probiotic products

Homofermenter	Facultative homofermenter	Obligate heterofermenter
Enterococcus faecium	*Lactobacillus bavaricus*	*Lactobacillus brevis*
E. faecalis	*L. casei*	*L. buchneri*
Lb. acidophilus	*L. coryniformis*	*L. cellobiosus*
L. lactis	*L. curvatus*	*L. confuses*
L. delbrueckii	*L. plantarum*	*L. coprophilus*
L. leichmannii	*L. sake*	*L. fermentatum*
L. salivarius		*L. sanfrancisco*
Streptococcus brevis		*Leuconostoc dextranicum*
S. thermophilus		*Leu. mesenteroides*
Ped. acidilactici		*Leu. Paramesenteroides*
P. damnosus		
P. pentosaceous		

Adapted from Prado *et al.*, (2008) and Leroy *et al.*, (2008).

Presently, probiotics are exclusively consumed as fermented dairy products, yogurt or freeze dried cultures (Douglas and Sanders, 2008). Novel modes of therapeutic and prophylactic interventions may include the consumption of probiotics either alone or in combination with prebiotics.

A prebiotic is a non-digestible food affecting the host beneficially by selectively stimulating the growth and activity of one or a limited number of bacteria in the colon. Prebiotics are particularly nondigestible oligosaccharides and fructo oligosaccharides naturally found in onions, garlic, leeks, chicory, artichokes, beans and peas. They are also present in some cereals. A mixture of prebiotics and probiotics is known as symbiotic. Here it beneficially affects the host by improving the survival and implantation of live microbial dietary supplements in the GIT ultimately improving the health of the host and its wellbeing. Harty *et al.* (1994) have studied the pathogenic potential of *Lactobacilli*.

2
PROBIOTIC PROPERTIES SELECTION AND BENEFITS

There are potential beneficial medicinal uses of probiotics for which research is limited and only preliminary results are available. Recent research on the molecular biology and genomics of *Lactobacillus* has focused on the interaction with the immune system, anti-cancer potential, and potential as a biotherapeutic agent in case of antibiotic-associated diarrhoea, traveller's diarrhoea, pediatric diarrhoea, inflammatory bowel diseases and irritable bowel syndrome (Ljungh *et al.*, 2009). Studies of some probiotics tested *in vitro* on human epithelial cell lines have shown that they could block the adhesion of shiga toxin producing *E. coli* (Sherman *et al.*, 2005). These are claimed to be health promoting and/or disease preventing beyond the basic function of supplying nutrients. Probiotic foods are emerging as an important category of food supplements. Earlier workers have shown the inhibition of diarrhea caused by *E.coli* using probiotic lactic acid bacteria and yeast (Yan and Polk, 2006). Ratledge *et al.* (2002) have studied the biochemistry and molecular biology of lipid accumulation in oleaginous microorganisms.

All effects can be attributed to the individual strain(s) tested. Testing of a supplement does not indicate benefit from any other strain of the same species, and testing does not indicate benefit from the whole group of LAB (or other probiotics) (Gilliland *et al.*, 1984b). Probiotic culture cannot exert beneficial effects unless their population reaches a certain level. They need to be viable, active and abundant in the concentration of at least log 10^6 cfu g^{-1} in the product throughout the specified shelf life (Vinderola *et al.*, 2000). All probiotic foods should be safe and have good sensory properties (Saarela *et al.*, 2000). Shobharani and Agrawal (2010) have studied the interception of quorum sensing signal molecule by furanone to enhance the shelf life of fermented milk. Levitt *et al.* (1995) have discussed the metabolism of gas formation in the large intestine due to colonic bacteria.

The viability of the culture is an important aspect in any functional food. Various methods have been used to improve the growth and survival of these probiotic bacteria during storage such as oligosaccharides, inulin (Cummings *et al.*, 2001), sugar sources (Carvalho *et al.*, 2003a), peptides and essential amino acids (Dave and Shah, 1998).

When milk was supplemented with a combination of protein hydrolysates, fructose whey protein concentrate, tomato juice and papaya pulp it was observed that the growth of *L. acidophilus* was improved. With cysteine, acid hydrolysate, tryptone, vitamins, dextrin and maltose an improvement in the viability of *Bifidobacteria* was seen. Prebiotics, such as oligosaccharides, are added to food, mainly to allow the preferential growth of probiotic organisms (Lourens-Hattingh and Viljoen, 2001).

Ascorbic acid is a highly effective antioxidant molecule. Small amounts of these molecules in the body can protect proteins, lipids, and nucleic acids from damage by free radicals and reactive oxygen species that are generated during normal metabolism and rapid growth. Ascorbic acid is water soluble, and not stored in the body, making regular intake necessary to prevent scurvy. The ascorbic acid content of food is strongly influenced by handling and storing practices (Bank *et al.*, 1985).

The selection of a suitable strain of a microorganism is regarded as the primary requirement for its use as a probiotic product.

The micro organisms used in probiotic preparations should be:

- Generally recognized as safe (GRAS) status
- Resistant to bile, hydrochloric acid and pancreatic juice
- Stimulate immune system
- Anti-carcinogenic
- Having reduced intestinal permeability
- Produce lactic acid
- Able to survive in both acidic conditions of the stomach and alkaline conditions of the duodenum (Vimala *et al.*, 2006).

Renu Agrawal *et al.* (2010) have studied the differences in biochemical and electrophoretic properties in *Lactobacillus plantarum*. They must be capable of producing antagonistic metabolites against a dominating saprophytic micro flora resulting in a competitive growth with a dose of 5 billion colony forming units a day (5×10^9 cfu/day) which has been recommended, for at least 5 days (Gupta and Garg, 2009).

An effective probiotic should exert a beneficial effect on the host, be non pathogenic and non-toxic, contain a large number of host cells, should have the ability to survive and metabolize in the gut, remain viable during storage, should be able to isolate from the same host as its intended host and should have good sensory properties. Marteau *et al.* (1997) studied in a dynamic system model of stomach and small intestine on the survivability of lactic acid bacteria. Marttinen *et al.* (2011) observed that short term consumption of probiotic did not affect the pH.

Adherence to the intestinal epithelial cells

The adhesion process of a probiotic involves different biophysical and biochemical properties between probiotics and epithelial cell layers. These include electrostatic interactions, passive and steric forces, hydrophobicity, autoaggregation capacity and specific cellular structures such as external appendages. These properties vary among the probiotic strains and are reported as species-specific characteristics (Schillinger *et al.*, 2005, Collado *et al.*, 2007; Randheera *et al.*, 2014). Probiotic need to survive the passage of the gastrointestinal tract and must be able to adhere and colonize the intestinal epithelium in order to compete with pathogenic organisms (Monteagudo *et al.*, 2012; Randheera *et al.*, 2014). This competition can result in removing the pathogenic microorganisms (Tuomola, 1999) which will reduce the risk of diseases arising from pathogenic organisms (Chapman *et al.*, 2014) and making this an important selection criterion. High adherence capacity was observed in the strains of *L. reuteri* which would enhance the epithelial barrier *in vitro* within 24 hours (Jensen *et al.*, 2012). Recently Argyri *et al.* (2013) found good adhesion ability of *L. pentosus* E108, *L. plantarum* B282 and *L. paracasei* sub sp. paracasei E94 to Caco-2 cells, 268. Greene and Klaenhammer (1994) studied the factors involved in adherence of *Lactobacilli* to human Caco-2 cells. Excellent adhesion properties of *P. pentosaceus* CIAL-86 were observed with anti-adhesion activity against *E. coli* CIAL-153 (García-Ruiz *et al.*, 2014). Inhibitory activities against *Campylobacter jejuni* were found with strains of *L. plantarum* N8, N9, ZL5 ZL4 and *L. casei*. It also inhibited the adhesion and invasion of HT-29 cells by *C. jejuni* (Wang *et al.*, 2014). Due to the adhesion ability of *Lactobacillus* strains as probiotics it was found that it promoted good residence time in the intestine, exclusion of pathogens and interaction with host cells to protect epithelial cells and it also induces immune modulation (Ouwehand *et al.*, 1999a). Schiffrin *et al.* (1997) studied the immuno modulation of blood leukocytes in humans by lactic acid bacteria as a criterion for selection of the strain.

The difficulties of studying bacterial adhesion *in vivo* led to the development of *in vitro* models for preliminary studies of adherent strains (Vesterlund *et al.*,

2007). Tests such as hydrophobicity and autoaggregation were performed as the cell surface traits have been considered necessary for adhesion. These traits facilitate temporary colonization as well as protection of the host system because of the biofilm formation over the host tissue. Some studies have shown that hydrophobicity and autoaggregation are important for promoting the colonization of probiotics in ecological niches such as the intestinal tract or the urogenital tract (Pelletier *et al.*, 1997; Del Re *et al.*, 2000; Giaouris *et al.*, 2009).

One of the physico-chemical properties in cell surface hydrophobicity is to facilitate the contact of microorganism and the host cells (Schillinger *et al.*, 2005). Physicochemical interactions mediate the initial and reversible contact stages including hydrophobicity which are thought to be nonspecific but play an important role (Pelletier *et al.*, 1997). Isolates that exhibit high hydrophobicity values also high capacity for autoaggregation and adherence to Caco-2 cells were studied (Kotzamanidis *et al.*, 2010). *Lactobacillus* that showed an affinity for an apolar solvent above 40% showed higher hydrophobic characteristics (Giaouris *et al.*, 2009). Dias *et al.* (2013) have reported that *Lactobacillus* strains have high hydrophobicity of 59% and 54.75%, respectively (Ren *et al.* 2014).

Adhesion autoaggregation and coaggregation of probiotics are important processes to the intestinal epithelium and barriers should be formed to prevent colonization by pathogenic microorganisms (Del Re *et al.*, 2000). For all cell adherence properties aggregation is a phenotype (Pelletier *et al.*, 1997; Kos *et al.*, 2003). Del Re *et al.* (2000) have shown that the strains which have values lower than 10% are non-autoaggregating. Strains of *L. salivarius* and *L. plantarum* have high autoaggregation capacity (Ren *et al.*, 2012). According to Ren *et al.* (2014) *L. salivarius* sub sp. *salicinius*, *L. acidophilus* and *L.plantarum* have high values for autoaggregation (46%, 45% and 34%, respectively) when it was compared with reference to *L. rhamnosus* strain (33%). Four isolates of *Lactobacillus* showed autoaggregation values higher than 90% (Bautista-Gallego *et al.*, 2013).

The coaggregation abilities of the *Lactobacillus* species with potential pathogens might prevent the colonization of the gut by pathogenic bacteria (Bao *et al.*, 2010). The percentage of coaggregation is strain-specific (Collado *et al.*, 2007). In general, *Lactobacilli* have a higher coaggregation with *Listeria monocytogenes* (Dias *et al.*, 2013) which may be related to the formation of mixed species biofilms. Vesterlund *et al.* (2005) studied the adhesion of bacteria to resected human colonic tissue. Duary *et al.* (2011) have assessed the adhesion on human colonic epithelial cells.

Antimicrobial activity of probiotics

Production of antimicrobial peptides is another important mechanism by which the probiotic bacterium contributes beneficially to its host. The first antimicrobial peptide was discovered by Gratia (1925) from gram negative bacteria called as colicins and those peptides from gram positive bacteria are called as bacteriocins.

Bacteriocins are proteinaceous antimicrobial compounds that are produced by bacteria and which usually inhibits the closely related species. Bacteriocins are low molecular weight peptides compared to colicins and do not possess a specific receptor for adsorption (Jack *et al.*, 1995). Rodriguez *et al.* (2000) have studied the diversity in bacteriocins produced by lactic acid bacteria which were isolated from raw milk.

Gram positive bacteriocins produced by lactic acid bacteria are membrane active compounds that increase the permeability of the cytoplasmic membrane (Jack *et al.*, 1995). The inhibitory activity of these bacteriocins varies. Some inhibit *Lactobacilli* and some are active against wider range of gram positive and gram negative bacteria as well as yeasts and molds (Nemcova, 1997).

Examples of bacteriocins produced by LAB

Nisin - *Lactobacillus lactis*

Leucocin - *Leuconostoc gelidium*

Pediocin A - *Pediococcus pentosaceus*

LAB commonly produces bacteriocins which are proteins and have bacteriocidal activity against pathogenic microorganisms. *Helicobacter pylori* are inhibited by *L.acidophilus* and *E.coli* O157:H7 by *Saccharomyces cerevisiae* sp. boulardii (Lorea *et al.*, 2001). Strains of *Bifidobacterium infantis* and *Lactobacillus salivarious* inhibited *Clostridium difficile* and *E.coli* (Lee *et al.*, 2003). *Pediococcus* sp. was shown to have activity against *Pseudomonas aeruginosa*, *Bacillus cereus* and *Staphylococcus aureus* (Jamuna and Jeevaratnam, 2004). Adhesion of *E.coli* K88 to porcine intestinal mucus was inhibited by *Enterococcus faecium* 18 C23 (Zin *et al.*, 2000). Feeding probiotic foods to rats have made it possible to understand the relationship between microbial population in the gut and health where probiotics topped the list (Svanberg, 1995). Probiotics are known to inhibit diarrhea (Oberhelman *et al.*, 1999). Castor oil induced diarrhea model is most widely used as an experimental model to study substances with anti-diarrheal properties. It induces severe secretary diarrhea within 3h (Chitme *et al.*, 2004). It is due to one of the castor oil ingredient ricinoleic acid which induces the secretion of prostaglandins E2 in the gut lumen and increases the secretion of water and electrolytes into the small intestine. *Lactobacillus* inhibitor production against *Escherichia coli* and coaggregation ability with uropathogens has been shown. The data indicated that the inhibitory effect was not due to bacteriophages or hydrogen peroxide. Strain GR-1 was found to coaggregate with *E. coli* ATCC 25922 in urine (Reid *et al.*, 1988). Dziuba and Dziuba (2014) have studied the milk protein derived bioactive peptides in dairy products. Giraffa (1995) have shown the anti Listeria factors in enterococcal bacteriocins in dairy technology. Munoz *et al.* (2012) have studied the role of fructooligosaccharides and its effect on bacteriocin production in *Lactobacillus* strains isolated from corn and molasses. Renu Agrawal and Shylaja Dharmesh (2011) have isolated an antishigella protein from *Pediococcus pentosaceous*. Wilson *et al.* (2003) have demonstrated that *proapoptotic* BH3 only proteins trigger membrane integration of prosurvival Bcl-w. Winton *et al.* (1999) looked into the modulation of apoptosis and mutation frequency in the small intestine.

Nutrient synthesis and bioavailability

The action of micro-organisms during the preparation of cultured foods or in the digestive tract has been shown to improve the quantity, availability and digestibility of some dietary nutrients. Fermentation of food with probiotics has shown to increase folic acid in yogurt, bifidus milk and kefir (Rajalakshmi and Vanaja 1967; Shahani and Chandan 1979; Deeth and Tamime 1981; Alm 1982). Vitamins like niacin and riboflavin levels were also increased in yogurt with fermentation (Deeth and Tamime 1981; Alm 1982). Lactic acid bacteria are known to release various enzymes and vitamins into the intestinal lumen. This exerts synergistic effects on digestion, alleviating symptoms of intestinal malabsorption and produces lactic acid, which lowers the pH of the intestinal content and helps to inhibit the development of invasive pathogens such as Salmonella spp. or strains of *E. coli* (Mallett *et al.*, 1989; Mack *et al.*, 1999). Bacterial enzymatic hydrolysis may enhance the bioavailability of protein and fat (Fernandes *et al.*, 1987) and increase the production of free amino acids, short chain fatty acids (SCFA) like lactic acid, propionic acid and butyric acid. When absorbed these SCFAs contribute to the available energy pool of the host and may protect against pathological changes in the colonic mucosa (Leopold and Eileler, 2000). They also help to maintain an appropriate pH in the colonic lumen, which is critical in the expression of many bacterial enzymes and carcinogen metabolism in the gut (Mallett *et al.*, 1989). Shobharani and Agrawal (2008) have studied the effect on cellular membrane fatty acids under stressed conditions of *Leuconostoc mesenteroides* sub sp. Dextranicum. Apart from nutrient synthesis, the action of microorganisms improve the digestibility of some dietary nutrients. Several lines of evidence show that the appropriate strain of lactic acid bacteria, in adequate amounts, can alleviate symptoms of lactose intolerance. *Streptococcus thermophilus*, *Lactobacillus bulgaricus* and other *Lactobacilli* used in fermented milk products deliver enough bacterial lactase to the intestine and stomach where lactose is degraded to prevent symptoms in lactase non persistent individuals (Kilara and Shahani 1975; Martini *et al*., 1991a,b). Fermentation by the culture should preserve and enhance the quality in order to beneficially alter the flavour of the food (Rivera-Espinoza and Gallardo-Navarro, 2010) thereby generating a higher added-value product.

Table 2: Beneficial properties of some probiotic bacteria

Bacteria	Probiotic effects	Properties	Use
Lactobacillus acidophilus (six major species) (Danone Newsletter Number 13,1997) • may prevent colon cancer • may prevent cholesterolemia	• may fight intestinal infection • reduces intestinal transit time	Survives GI transit well (Ability to survive varies between strains.) Adherence demonstrated *in vitro* but not yet demonstrated *in vivo*.	Used in acidophilus milk and in kefir, may be used in yoghurt.
	A single strain of *L.acidophilus* will probably not accomplish all the supposed benefits.	Grows slowly in fermented products and doesn't survive much in fermented products.	
Lactobacillus GG (NutritionToday Supplement, No. 6, 1996)	• prevents growth of pathogens • delays tumor development • prevents traveller's diarrhea, antibiotic-associated bacteria, and infant diarrhea	Implants and colonizes the intestinal tract. Colonization not permanent.	Some new fermented dairy products using LGG are available in Europe. Minimum levels necessary for colonization are 10^8 cells in milk, 10^9 cells in fermented milk or enteric tablets, 10^{10} cells in gelatin capsules.

Adapted from Holzapfel *et al*., 2001

Selection of probiotics

The selection criteria for lactic acid bacteria to be used as probiotic include the following ability to:

- Exert a beneficial effect on the host
- Withstand into a foodstuff at high cell counts, and remain viable throughout

- The shelf-life of the product
- Withstand transit through the GI tract
- Adhere to the intestinal epithelium
- Cell lining and colonize the lumen of the tract
- Produce antimicrobial substances towards pathogens and
- Stabilize the intestinal microflora and be associated with health benefits.

Probiotics must have a good shelf life in food or preparations, containing a large number of viable cells at the time of consumption, and be non-pathogenic and nontoxic in their preparation. The most extensively studied and widely used probiotics are the lactic acid bacteria, particularly the *Lactobacillus* and *Bifidobacterium* spp.

Role of fatty acids in Lactic acid Bacteria

Fatty acids play a crucial role in the selection of probiotic strain. Oleic acid inhibits the mutagenic activity (Mensink *et al.* (2003) and it also reduces the risk of coronary heart disease (Hayatsu *et al.*, 1981), linoleic acid inhibits the initiation of carcinogenesis (Ha *et al.*, 1987; Pariza and Hargraves, 1985) and tumorigenesis activity in rats (Ip *et al.*, 1991). Yadav *et al.* (2007) reported that the gas chromatographic analysis of fatty acids have shown that the total free fatty acid increased during fermentation and storage periods in both probiotic and control dahi. The conjugated linoleic acid was found to increase in probiotic dahi samples during fermentation and it remained constant until 10 days of storage. Jhonson *et al.* (1995) reported that the LAB strains mainly produced cellular fatty acids like myristic, palmitic, hexadecenoic acid, stearic acid, oleic acid, cis-vaccenic, and dihydrosterculic acids. The strains grown without Tween 80 did not have oleic and dihydrosterculic acids among the cellular fatty acids. This indicates that oleic acid was not synthesized by the LAB strains. When the growth medium was supplemented with Tween 80, two new fatty acids (oleic acid and dihydrosterculic acid) were produced. Ayad *et al.* (1999) have shown the production of aldehyde, 2-methyl-1-propanol, 2-methyl-1-butanol from valine in certain strains of *Lactococci*. *Bifidobacterium* spp. produced short chain fatty acids with antimicrobial activity (Ip *et al.*, 1991). Jhonson *et al.* (1990) studied the microbiological safety of cheese made from heat-treated milk.

Short chain fatty acids are known to have therapeutic value. Caprylic acid is known to have antimicrobial properties (Alonso *et al.*, 2003; Ayad *et al.*, 1999; Ha *et al.*, 1987; Ip *et al.*, 1991; Kankaanpaa *et al.*, 2004; Martley and Crow,

1993). Lauric acid is known to have antibacterial function (Nakatsuji *et al.*, 2009; Drake *et al.*, 2008). Oleic acid inhibited the mutagenic activity (Drici-Cachon *et al.*, 1996) and also reduces the risk of coronary artery disease (Goldberg and Eschar, 1977). Initiation of carcinogenesis and tumorigenesis activity in rat was inhibited by conjugated linoleic acid (Endo *et al.*, 2006). Reddy (1998) have explained the rising burden of cardiovascular diseases in India.

3
CLASSIFICATION OF PROBIOTICS

LAB constitutes a group of gram positive bacteria. They are nonsporulating, nonrespiring but aerotolerant cocci or rods, which produce lactic acid as one of the main fermentation products of carbohydrates, they do not have cytochromes. They belong to the phylum Firmicuttes, class *Bacilli* and order *Lactobacillaceae*. The group includes several genera such as *Lactobacillus, Lactococcus, Bifidobacterium, Pediococcus, Enterobacter, Corynebacterium, Streptococcus, Leuconostoc* etc.

According to the Garitty *et al.*, in Bergey's Manual 2nd. Edition (2001), the genera that fulfil the description of LAB include:

- *Aerococcus*
- *Lactobacillus*
- *Leuconostoc*
- *Pediococcus*
- *Streptococcus*

Present system of Lactic acid bacteria classification

The current classification of lactic acid bacteria is based on analysis and sequencing of 16S rRNA (Olsen *et al.*, 1994). Bacteria are divided into branches namely Actinomycetes and *Clostridium* based on the content of G+C. The former has G+C content of more than 50 mol%. The genera that are included in this branch are *Bifidobacterium, Corynebacterium* and *Propionibacterium*. The latter contains below 50 mol% of G+C content and has the genera *Lactobacillus, Lactococcus, Leuconostoc, Pediococcus* and *Streptococcus*.

L.lactis has been isolated from milk, milk products, vegetables, fruits and cereal sources (Grahn, 1994; Lilliana and Stouvenel, 2006; Kimito, 2000; Kimito *et al.*,

2004; Kelly *et al.*, 1998). Adaptation to low pH and high concentrations of bile salts is important for lactic acid bacteria to survive in the GIT. The hind gut is the most heavily colonized and metabolically active organ of the body. Colon region harbours around 500 species of bacteria that are involved in fermenting the foods and in releasing bioactive compounds (Conway, 1995). Once the bacterium reaches the intestinal tract, their ability to survive depends on their resistance to bile (Gilliland *et al.*, 1984b). The survival rate of bacteria goes down when bile enters the duodenal region of the small intestine. Since bacterial cell membranes consist of lipids and fatty acids it is susceptible to destruction by bile salts. *Lactobacillus* sp. can hydrolyze bile salts (Jacobsen *et al.*, 1999; Lee and Salminen, 1995). Bile salt hydrolase activity deconjugates bile salts and protects the bacteria from toxicity. Bacterial attachment to the epithelial wall of the ileum controls the intestinal flora of that region, which may be a defense mechanism against the colonization of the small intestine by undesirable bacteria from the caecum (Sarra *et al.*, 1992). Gismondo *et al.* (1999) have written a review article on effect of probiotics to modify gastrointestinal flora. De Smet (1995) has studied the significance of bile salt hydrolase activity of *Lactobacilli*. Kos *et al.* (2003) reported that *L. acidophilus* M92 showed strong adherence to the ileal epithelial cell. When there is oxidation of lipids in foods it gives off-flavours and undesirable chemical compounds detrimental to health. Tannock *et al.* (1989) have discussed the role of *Lactobacilli* and bile salt hydrolase in the murine intestinal tract. When the culture has all these properties it is classified under LAB (lactic acid bacteria).

Yeasts reproduce primarily by budding and occasionally by fission and are eukaryotic unicellular fungi (Walker, 2009). They are characterized by a wide dispersion in natural habitats but most are frequently isolated from substrate with high amount of sugar, salt and low pH, temperature and water activity (Arroyo-lopez *et al.*, 2008). Yeasts are well known for their enormous importance in food and beverage production and they have been reported to be involved in the fermentation of several types of indigenous fermented foods and beverages (Jespersen, 2003). Among antibiotic resistance, vancomycin resistance is of major concern as vancomycin is a broad spectrum antibiotic and is used against clinical infection caused by multi drug resistant pathogens (Johnson *et al.*, 1990; Woodford *et al.*, 1995). The resistance of the culture to vancomycin is usually dangerous because it can spread the drug resistant pathogenic cultures causing incurable diseases. Erdogrul and Erbilir (2006) reported *L. bulgaricus* to be sensitive to vancomycin.

4
DISEASES KNOWN TO BE INHIBITED BY PROBIOTICS

4a. Intestinal Disorders

History of health claims

According to Bottazzi (1983) it was in 76 BC that the Roman historian Plinius recommended the use of fermented milk for treating gastroenteritis. Metchnikoff claimed that the intake of fermented milk containing *Lactobacilli* reduces the toxin producing bacteria, thereby increasing the longetivity of the host (Metchnikoff, 1908). Tissier (1905) showed that there was an increase in the *Bifidobacteria* in breast fed-infants, thus claiming that the administration of *Bifidobacteria* to infants suffering from diarrhea was very beneficial as they supersede the putrefactive bacteria that causes the disease. Intestinal beneficial microfloras are responsible to resist the disease (Bohnhoff *et al*., 1954).

Disturbance of homeostatic control results in diarrhea, inflammation and various intestinal diseases. Homeostatis depends on the equilibrium between absorption (nutrients, ions) secretion (ions, IgA) and barrier capacity (to pathogens and macromolecules) of the digestive epithelium.

There can be dysregulation of ion coupled nutrient absorption. With an abnormal stimulation of ion secretion the water loss increases. Water movement is due to sodium solute co transport systems of (Na^+ glucose) or (Cl^-) secretion across the apical membranes of intestinal epithelial cells.

Chloride secretion affects electrolyte and water movements. Pathogenic bacteria adhere to brush border membranes of the enterocyte, including epithelial dysfunction as lesions and release of toxins or cytotoxins disrupting epithelial integrity (Ng *et al*., 2008, Heyman and Menard, 2002). Osmotic diarrhea can be induced when a non-absorbable compound (lactose) reaches the intestinal lumen.

Abnormal stimulation of the underlying immune system may lead to the release of inflammatory mediators which have the ability to alter epithelial function (Heyman and Menard, 2002).

Today the use of probiotics and prebiotics as therapeutic agents for GI disorders is moving into main stream therapy (deVrese *et al.*, 2005). Shobha rani and Agrawal (2011) have isolated and characterized a potent probiotic lactic acid bacteria strain from cheddar cheese with antimicrobial property. Chen *et al.* (2005) have looked into the reference data base for virulence factor in bacteria. Saavendra *et al.* (1994) have found beneficial effects in infants by feeding probiotics.

4a.1 Diarrhea

Several types of diarrhea can be prevented by lactic acid bacteria (Sanders, 1994). Fermented milk products are known to effectively prevent or treat infantile diarrhea which have been verified by a number of well-designed studies (Saloff-Coste, 1995). Effects have been noted with *L. casei* and *B. bifidum*. Lactic acid bacteria can reduce antibiotic-related diarrhea (Salminen and Deighton, 1992). Lactic acid bacteria have a role in immunosuppressed patients who use antibiotics routinely (Aronsson *et al.*, 1987).

Effectiveness of lactic acid bacteria in decreasing the incidence of traveller's diarrhea has been demonstrated (Black *et al.*, 1989). Lactic acid bacteria can probably reduce diarrhea in several ways:

- Competition with pathogens for nutrients and space in the intestine (Salminen and Deighton, 1992).
- A direct effect against the pathogens is by the formation of by-products. *In vitro* studies have shown that and *L.bulgaricus L.casei, L.acidophiluscan* all produce antimicrobial agents such as acidophilin and bulgarican that can inhibit growth of pathogens (Salminen and Deighton, 1992).
- Effects on the immune system may be effective against diarrhea.

Diarrhea is caused due to different pathogens. Presently, there are many studies done in this regard and there are evidences that probiotics have beneficial effects on many different types of diarrhea. In the treatment of rotavirus diarrhea, *Lactobacillus* GG is reported to be effective (Pant *et al.*, 1996; Guandalini *et al.*, 2000). Also *Lactobacillus acidophilus* LB1, *Bifidobacterium lactis* and *Lactobacillus* reuteri are reported to have beneficial effects (Salminen *et al.*, 2001). Another type of diarrhea is traveler's diarrhea which affects the healthy traveller's. Oksanen *et al.* (1990) evaluated the efficacy of *Lactobacillus* GG in preventing diarrhea in 820 people travelling from Finland to Turkey. Antibiotic associated diarrhea is another type which is very common. Due to the suppression of normal microflora during the microbial therapy it results in more pathogenic strains. The main reason for antibiotic associated diarrhea (AAD) is due to the resistant strains of *Clostridium difficile*.

Antibiotic-associated diarrhea

Antibiotic-associated diarrhea (AAD) results from an imbalance in the colonic microbiota caused by antibiotic therapy. Microbiota alteration, changes the carbohydrate metabolism with decreased short-chain fatty acid absorption and as a result osmotic diarrhea is developed. Another consequence of antibiotic therapy leading to diarrhea is overgrowth of potentially pathogenic organisms such as *Clostridium difficile*.

Probiotic treatment can reduce the incidence and severity of AAD as indicated in several meta-analyses (Rajkumar *et al.*, 2002; Cremonini *et al.*, 2002; Mcfarland, 2006; Szajewska *et al.*, 2006; Szymanski *et al.*, 2006; Sazawal *et al.*, 2006). However, further documentation of these findings through randomized, double blind, placebo-controlled trials are required to be done.

Efficacy of probiotic AAD prevention is dependent on the probiotic strain(s) used and on the dosage (Doron, 2008; Surawic, 2008). A reduction of 50% in AAD occurrence has been found (Sazawal *et al.*, 2006). No side-effects have been reported in any of these studies. It is important to check while administering probiotic supplements to immuno compromised individuals or patients who have a compromised barrier reducing inflammation.

AAD (Antibiotic associated diarrhea)

Around 20% of the patients under antibiotic treatment suffer from AAD due to the alterations in gut microflora which results in disturbances in intestinal carbohydrate or even in the metabolism of bile acid. Using Lb. GG a placebo trial was run and it was obsereved that there was a reduction of 25% (Bergogne-Berezin, 2000). Large decrease in AAD associated patients was seen by using multi strain probiotic milk (Mcfarland *et al.*, 1995 and Mcfarland, 2006). Probiotics are known to modulate the intestinal microflora (Madden *et al.*, 2005).

Radiotherapy-induced diarrhea

To cancer patients usually radiotherapy is given. Sometimes, it may injure the intestine which reduces the absorption and translocation of bacteria. It was seen that the side effects were reduced with *L. acidophilus* and *L. rhamnosus* in such patients (Urbancsek *et al.*, 2001).

Clostridium difficile associated diarrhea

In USA 15-20% patients get *C.difficile* associated diarrhea due to antibiotics. Mc Farland *et al.* (1994) and Mc Farland (2006) examined a therapy to patients with *S.boulardii* and found significant inhibition in the disease along with antibiotics.

Traveller's diarrhea

Traveller's diarrhea is commonly caused by enterotoxigenic *Escherichiacoli*. For this double blind, randomized controlled trials suggested preventive efficacy of LGG and *S.boulardii* (Mc Farland, 2007). Black *et al.* (1989) have shown the prophylactic efficacy of *Lactobacilli* on traveller's diarrhea.

Infantile diarrhea

This is caused by Rotavirus where the intestinal permeability increases simultaneously increasing the levels of beta-lactoglobulin which contains immune complexes (Chouraqui *et al.*, 2008). Recently, in a double blind, placebo controlled trial, administration of LGG to infants with diarrhea reduced the duration (Szymanski *et al.*, 2006).

HIV/AIDS associated diarrhea

Human immunodeficiency virus (HIV) infection also causes diarrhea (Rolfe, 2000). There is no effective therapy for this disease. However when probiotics were fed the CD4 counts were higher in number in probiotic fed patients. The probiotics are known to have immune stimulatory properties which can also treat children infected with HIV (Trois *et al.*, 2008).

Enteral Feeding associated diarrhea

Due to a change in the normal flora and during metabolism of carbohydrate diarrhea is developed on nasogastric tube feeding in the patients. Bleichner *et al.* (1997) found that it could be prevented by feeding of *S. boulardii* culture.

Chronic diarrhea

Acute diarrhea becomes chronic if it lasts for more than two weeks. Feeding of fermented milk to children has shown to eliminate the disease in 4 days in patients suffering with post gastroenteritis syndrome (Gonzalez *et al.*, 1994).

4a.2 BSH (Bile Salt hydrolase) activity

In Vivo studies

Lactic acid bacteria with high BSH activity lower the serum cholesterol levels through an interaction with the host bile salt metabolism (De Smet *et al.*, 1994). De Smet *et al.* (1998) studied the effects of feeding live *Lactobacillus reuteri* cells containing active bile salt hydrolase (BSH) on plasma cholesterol levels in pigs. Cholesterol removal from culture media was a result of precipitation of cholesterol with free bile acids, due to the activity of the bacterial enzyme bile salt hydrolase (Klaver and Van der Meer, 1993). Kim *et al.* (2008) studied the factors responsible for the cholesterol reduction by *Lactobacillus acidophilus* ATCC 43121. The results showed that the cell-free supernatant (CFS) produced by ATCC 43121 along with bile salts could reduce cholesterol in the broth also.

4a.3 Helicobacter pylori Infection

Chronic gastritis and peptic ulcer are caused by *H. pylori* which has a risk for gastric malignancies (Lesbros-Pantoflickova *et al.*, 2007). Probiotics have shown positive effects and can be used as a prophylactic therapy (Sabbi *et al.*, 2008).

LAB'S are also utilized in the treatment of *Helicobacter pylori* infections (which cause peptic ulcers) in adults. Presently the probiotic cultures are used in combination with standard medical treatments. However, more studies are required to be done in this area (Hamilton, 2003).

4a.4 Tumor

Promising results are shown by lactic acid bacteria against stomach ulcers. Work with a specific strain of *L. acidophilus* demonstrated that *L. acidophiluscompetes* effectively (*in vitro*) against *Helicobacter pylori* for attachment sites, limiting the number of *H. pylori* that can attach to the cell wall (Brassart, 1995). Infection with *H. pylori* may cause stomach ulcers. A study of patients with ulcers showed that *Bifidobacterium bifidum* promoted healing of gastric ulcers in 50% of the patients and eradication of *H. pylori* from the mucous membranes in 30% of the patients (Lee and Salminen, 1995). Sabbi *et al.* (2005) have shown inhibition of *Helicobacter pylori* by using probiotics in infants.

According to Prieto *et al.* (2012) trophic effects were seen by probiotic strains which included improvement of the bioavailability of nutrients and the production of functionally and nutritionally desirable metabolites *in vivo*, including specific enzymes, proteins, fatty acids and vitamins. Probiotic strains are able to secrete digestive enzymes (amylase, lipase and protease) to complement those secreted in the host intestine (Grady and Gibson, 2007). Probiotics are carrier of the enzymes that are deficient but essential to aid availability of nutrients in the intestine. Probiotic strains which have high phytase activity improve the bioavailability of iron and zinc, which are important micronutrients in diets but largely unavailable for uptake in the human intestine, which lack digestive phytase (Hellström *et al.*, 2010). Yeasts are eukaryotic unicellular microfungi that asexually reproduce primarily by budding or fission, and do not form their sexual states (spores) in or on a fruiting body (Walker, 2009; Kurtzman *et al.*, 2011). Mostly they are obligate aerobes however; some are facultative anaerobes also (Bamforth, 2005). Yeasts are broadly categorized into two phyla within the fungi kingdom, the ascomycetes and basidiomycetes (Jacques and Casaregola, 2008). Ascomycetous yeasts form ascospores inside the cell, while basidiomycetous yeasts develop external spores. Yeasts have ultrastructural features similar to that of higher eukaryotic cells (Walker, 2009). The cell wall consists of β-1, 3 glucan which makes up about 50% of cell wall dry weight and chitin with 1-2% of cell wall dry weight which are mostly present in the inner layer. β-1, 6glucan (8% of cell wall dry weight) and various mannoproteins (40-50% of cell wall dry weight) are present in the outer layer (Gunasekaran *et al.*, 2012). Corsetti *et al.* (1998) reported a strain of *L. sanfrancisco* CB1, isolated from sourdough which produced caproic acid and played a key role in the inhibitory activity against bacteria and mould. Propionic acid, butyric acid and valeric acid are responsible for antifungal activity. Conjugated linoleic acid (CLA) is potentially very beneficial for improving biological effects and has gained considerable importance. CLA composition inhibits the initiation of carcinogenesis (Devery *et al.*, 2001; Pariza *et al.*, 2001). Kankaanpaa *et al.* (2004) reported that in *L.rhamnosus*, *L.casei* and *L.delbrueckii* when polyunsaturated fatty acids such as linoleic, α-linolenic acid, γ-linolenic acid, arachidonic and docosahexanoic acids were added to the growth medium affected the fatty acid composition of total lipids.

The most interesting role of antioxidants, both biologically and technologically is the interaction with oxidative free radicals. Pyo *et al.* (2005) studied the antioxidative activity of probiotic lactic acid bacteria (LAB) and *Bifidobacterium* in *in vivo* experiments using rats that were deficient in vitamin E (Kaizu *et al.*, 1993). Lin and Yen (1999) studied the antioxidative property of (19) LAB strains. Gayathri and Agrawal (2012) have studied the antioxidant activity and fatty acid profile of fermented milk prepared by *Pediococcus pentosaceus* from different sources. Most of the strains tested demonstrated excellent reducing activity. In another investigation, the strain of *L. plantarum* containing high intracellular manganese was found to be more resistant to the oxygen dependent toxicity (Frederick and Fridovich, 1981). Mishra *et al.* (2012)

estimated the antiradical properties of antioxidants using DPPH assay: A critical review by sanders (1995) has reported the stress response in *L. lactis* by cloning, expression analysis and mutation of the Lactococcal superoxide dismutase gene.

Ito *et al.* (2001) studied the antioxidative effects of live *Bifidobacteria* on lipid peroxidation in the colonic mucosa of rats. It was found that the level of lipid peroxide decreased depending on bacterial concentration in the colonic mucosa. Oral administration of *B. bifidum* strain for two weeks significantly decreased the level of lipid peroxide in the colonic mucosa of iron overloaded mice (Ito *et al.*, 2003). Mishra *et al.* (2012) estimated the antiradical properties of antioxidants using DPPH assay in a review article.

Kullisar *et al.* (2003) studied the effect of fermented goat's milk with *Lactobacillus* fermentum ME-3 on antiatherogenicity in healthy subjects. They also reported that the prolonged resistance of lipoprotein fraction to oxidation and a lowered level of peroxidized lipoproteins were demonstrated.

4a.5 Bowel

It is difficult to determine any chronic colon problem that causes Irritable bowel syndrome (IBS). The disease causes symptoms like diarrhea, constipation, alternating diarrhea, excess intestinal gas, intestinal cramping, and bowel movements which are very severe. There is a mucous discharge from the rectum. Following meals there is abdominal discomfort and presence of stool in the colon. A double-blind placebo-controlled trial was done having constipation-predominant irritable bowel syndrome. Participants were given either placebo or a probiotic formula containing *Bifidobacterium animalis*. The results in the study period showed that use of the probiotic led to a significant reduction in discomfort of the colon compared to placebo. Probiotic EcN shows effects in irritable bowel syndrome, especially in patients with altered enteric microflora, e.g. after gastroenterocolitis or administration of antibiotics. The probiotic treatment increased the stool frequency very significantly. Probiotics are recommended after every use of antibiotic (Kruis *et al.*, 2012). Sergio (2001) have studied the use of *Bacillus* culture when given orally for the improvement of gastro intestinal problems.

4a.6 HIV

Lactobacillus rhamnosus GR-1 is known for good survival in milk (Hekmat and Reid, 2007; Hekmat and Soltani 2009) and it can be supplemented into yogurt (Hekmat and Reid, 2006; Baroja *et al.*, 2013) which gives a good taste and texture simultaneously (Hekmat and Reid, 2006). Earlier it was shown that this strain when added to yogurt was able to enhance immunity (Baroja *et al.*, 2013) and reduce the levels of diarrhea in HIV patients.

Before starting consumption, the 68 yogurt consumers had experienced an average increase in CD4 count of 0.16 cells/µl/day. After consumption of probiotic yogurt an additional increase of CD 4 to 0.28 cells/µl/day was observed. When adjusting for length of time using ART medication, this remained 0.17 cells/µl/day. The additional CD4 increase during the first 70 days was 0.73 CD4 cells/µl/day and this continued to rise. After this initial period the CD4 count continued to rise at 0.2 CD4 cells/µl/day.

4a.7 Lactase deficiency

Sucrase isomaltase deficiency

Usually carbohydrates are utilized by bacteria as a source of energy for growth, replication and metabolic processes. They can use many different sources of carbohydrates, some of the most common are glucose, fructose, pentose and lactose. Probiotic bacteria mostly include all lactic acid bacteria, which includes *Lactobacilli*, *Bifidobacteria* and *Streptococci*. Most of these lactic acid bacteria use glucose as their primary energy source, an exception being *Streptococcus thermophillus* which uses lactose preferentially (Kim and Gilliland, 1983). Most of the lactic acid bacteria primarily ferment glucose however utilization of lactose has been observed (Rorick and Scrimshaw, 1979).

For lactose metabolism it is important to have intracellular transport system allowing them to take up lactose and it should have the ability to produce the enzyme β-galactosidase (also known as lactase). This enzyme breaks down lactose into β-galactose and glucose, which can be metabolised to produce energy (Hove *et al.*, 1994).

Lactose metabolism

For lactose utilization as energy source the bacterial strain must be able to ingest the sugar and take it to the part of the cell which produces lactase where the lactose is broken into its composite parts by the enzyme. β-galactose and glucose are then metabolised via different pathways to produce energy. These different metabolic processes are known to produce many energetic molecules, in the form of ATP and a number of other molecules like lactate, ethanol and carbon dioxide.

Similar intracellular transport mechanism is taken up in *Lactobacillus acidophilus*, *Lactobacillus bulgaricus* and *Lactobacillus rhamnosus* as also in *Bifidobacterium* species to metabolize lactose. However, they produce different molecules during the metabolism to produce energy. *Lactobacillus casei* and *Streptococcus thermophilus* use a different method to move lactose into the right part of the cell as lactose phosphate. This produces the same metabolic products as the other *Lactobacillus* species (Almeida, 2012). Bacterial adaptation to lactase deficiency has been studied (Hill, 1983). The role of galactosidase in lactose metabolism is well studied by Devrese *et al*. (1992, 1995).

Lactose Maldigestion and Intolerance

Lactase insufficiency is caused due to low concentration of the lactose-cleaving enzyme β-galactosidase situated in the brush border membrane of the mucosa of the small intestine. Due to this, digestion of the disaccharide lactose is not enough causing lactose malabsorption (Bayless, 1981). Lactose maldigestion is due to an increase in blood glucose concentration of <1.12 mmol/L. In addition to intestinal lactase activity it is important to know the age and gender (Deshpandeetal., 2007). Dietary components taken along with lactose (meal effect), the rate of gastric emptying, the transit time in the gastrointestine and interactions among these factors (Vesa *et al*., 1997). Around the globe the prevalence of primary lactose maldigestion is 3-5% in Scandinavia, 17% in Finland, 5-15% in Great Britain, 15% in Germany, 15-20% in Austria, 17% in northern France, 65% in southern France, 20-70% in Italy, 55% in the Balkans, 70-90% in Africa (exeptions: Bedouins, 25%; Tuareg, 13%; Fulani, 22%), 80% in Central Asia, 90-100% in Eastern Asia, 30% in northern India, 70% in southern India, 15% in North American whites, 80% in North American blacks, 53% in North American Hispanics, and 65-75% in South America (Sahi, 1994; Johnson, 1981). Lactose maldigestion may occur in different forms. In adults lactose malabsorption is high at birth, which is low in childhood and adolescence. Lactase nonpersistence is normal in mammals and humans (Sieber *et al*., 1997). With the exception of the population of Northern and Central Europe and in America and Australia, 70-100% of adults worldwide are lactose malabsorbers. Predominant primary lactase deficiency is among the ages of 2 to 6 years. Among the white population the prevalence of lactase maldigestion starts later, this in some cases is after adulthood (20y). The frequencies of lactose maldigestion at ages 2 to 3y, 6y, and 9 to 10y, respectively, are 0%, 0%, and 6% in white Americans; 18%, 30%, and 47% in Americans of Mexican descent; 25%, 45%, and 60% in black South Africans; 30%, 80%, and 85% in Chinese and Japanese; and 30-55%, 90%, and >90% in Mestizos of Peru (Sahi, 1994; Woteki, 1976). Vogelsang *et al*. (1987) has written an article on lactose intolerance. Woteki *et al*. (1976) have studied the lactose malabsorption in Mexican American children.

Inflammation or functional loss of the small intestinal mucosa (enteritis, morbus Crohn, bacterial or parasitic infections, and bowel syndrome) or malnutrition may be the cause for secondary lactose malabsorption. Although some forms are transient, disappearing after recovery from the original disease, others are irreversible (Vogelsang, 1987). Congenital lactose malabsorption, a rare autosomal-recessive heritable genetic defect has been observed immediately after birth. Afflicted newborns respond to their first milk feed with diarrhea (Johnson, 1981). Montanarai *et al.* (2000) have studied the mechanism of how beta galactosidase is released from *Lactobacilli*.

Lactase maldigestion along with clinical symptoms like bloating, flatulence, nausea, diarrhea, and abdominal pain is termed as lactose in tolerance. Symptoms are caused by undigested lactose in the large intestine, where the lactose serves as a fermentable substrate for the bacterial flora and osmotically increases water flow into the lumen. The amount of lactose ingested causes the extent of symptoms. It also depends on individual sensitivity, the rate of gastric emptying, gastrointestinal transit time, and the pattern of microflora in the large intestine after the application of antibiotics. All this shows that lactose maldigestion is different from lactose intolerance (Vesa, 1997).

Lactose-intolerant people can ingest a certain amount of lactose without having adverse symptoms. Most of these people tolerate e > 9-12 g (equivalent to 200 mL or 1 glass of milk) (Johnson, 1981; Johnson *et al.*, 1994). Newcomer *et al.* (1978) found no significant difference in tolerance in American Indians (9% of subjects with symptoms) who were provided with 0-18g lactose. Most lactose malabsorbers tolerate 0.5-7.0 g lactose without symptoms of intolerance. Lactose in milk or yogurt has been found to be tolerated in persons undergoing jejunostomy where lactose maldigestion takes place (Arrigoni *et al.*, 1994).

A data on the prevalence of lactose maldigestion and the proportion of lactose-intolerant people within the malabsorber population segment in Germany were assessed. Healthy male and female volunteers aged 18-36y and living in northern Germany were screened with use of the breath-hydrogen test. To avoid over- or under representation of participants who classified themselves as milk intolerant or lactose malabsorbing, whole groups were tested, eg; all the employees of a department or all the students of a class were taken into consideration. Some 202 subjects took part in the screening. Of these 29 (14.4%) were maldigesters as proven by an increase of breath hydrogen >20 ppm after the ingestion of 25 g lactose on 3 consecutive occasions. Abdominal bloating, flatulence, and borborygmi are probably caused by gaseous products of lactose fermentation, such as hydrogen, CH_4, and carbon dioxide. Theoretically, <17 L of hydrogen are produced microbially from 50g lactose in the colon (Suarez *et al.*, 1995). If allowed to accumulate, this volume would have major implications for intestinal distension and gas problems. However, most of this gas is consumed by other intestinal bacteria. Surprisingly, subjects complaining of excessive gas in the gut had the same degree of lactose maldigestion and the same gas production as did subjects without complaints, although the former showed that the intestinal motility was not in order and this increased pain response to gut distension. When the same volumes of gas were actively infused into the intestine of these patients, the gases caused much more discomfort and had a greater tendency to reflux back into the stomach than was the case in control experiments with healthy subjects (Hammer *et al.*, 1996; Lasser *et al.*, 1975). Subjective (Psychological) discomfort (Mc Bean and Miller, 1998) of the intestine (eg, irritable bowel syndrome) (Vesa *et al.*, 1998) may be wrongly related to milk consumption by the subjects themselves. Martini *et al.* (1987) studied the effect of lactose digestion in yoghurt galactosidase. Sieber *et al.* (1997) have discussed the lactose intolerance by consuming milk.

Correlation between lactose maldigestion and symptoms of intolerance

A correlation has been found between lactose maldigestion and symptoms of lactose intolerance. Lactose reduction or improvement in lactose digestion indirectly improves gastrointestinal symptoms. Owing to the complex interplay of causative factors, lactose maldigestion does not correlate well with the symptoms of lactose intolerance. Only some of the lactose maldigesters have been found to be lactose intolerant. Manifestations of clinical symptoms occur much later after the decline of lactase activity. It is important to know that lactose-free diets do not cure the symptoms of all lactose-intolerant cases (Onwulata, 1989; Briet *et al.*, 1997). Savaiano (2011) have discussed the risk of low bone density due to lactose intolerance and how it can be improved with milk and milk products.

It is generally accepted that fermented milk products like yogurt can efficiently improve lactose digestion (Kolars *et al.*, 1984). Lactose digestion studies show better results in lactose malabsorbers when they consume nonheated yogurt rather than milk or pasteurized yogurt (Gilliland and Kim, 1983).

Malabsorption of sucrose causes hydrogen to get accumulated in the colon which results in diarrhea. *S.cerevisiae* along with sucrose has been found to prevent the same (Harms *et al.*, 1987). Lactose is sometimes not digested due to the deficiency of lactase. Probiotic bacteria like *L.acidophilus* and *Bifidobacteria* produce β-d-galactosidase which digets lactose (Vesa *et al.*, 1996, 1998).

It is well-known that the presence of lactic acid bacteria, specifically *L. bulgaricus* and *S. thermophilus* in yoghurt, improves lactose digestion (Martini *et al.*, 1991a). It appears that the cell walls of the bacteria have to be intact (as is the case when the bacteria are alive) for the positive effect to happen (Kuhn, 1996). Some possible mechanisms for the improved lactose digestion include:

- In the intestine lactase digests the lactose (Martini *et al.*, 1987).
- The slower transit time of yoghurt may permit more time for the residual intestinal lactase and the bacteria in the yoghurt to digest lactose (Schaafsma, 1993).
- Something in the yoghurt may inhibit fermentation of lactose and thus reduce symptoms (Schaafsma, 1993).

For the digestion of lactose an essential enzyme β-galactosidase is required. In its absence lactose intolerant people cannot metabolize lactose. It has been noticed that after weaning a large number of population become lactose intolerant. Gilliland *et al.* (1989) has explained that β-galactosidase is an intracellular enzyme. As milk has lactose some people are notable to digest it. This is due to insufficient β-galactosidase to digest lactose in the intestine.

In many cases it has been found that the consumption of milk causes symptoms like abdominal pain, bloating, flatulence, cramping and diarrhoea. When certain starter cultures were added to the milk products it was found that it degrades lactose (Lin *et al.*, 1991; Scheinbach, 1998; Ouwehand and Salminen, 1998; Fooks *et al.*, 1999). The probiotics impart beneficial effects as it has high lactase enzyme which can act on lactose intolerant individuals (Salminen *et al.*, 2003). The products which have probiotic bacteria are quite efficient for lactose intolerant humans. It can withstand low pH and is able to improve digestibility of lactose by β-galactosidase production. No correlation exists to show relation between lactose maldigestion and the incidence of symptoms of intolerance, which include flatulence, abdominal pain, and diarrhea. It appears that probiotic baceria acts either by preventing symptoms of intolerance in the large intestine or by improving lactose digestion in the small intestine. When lactose is not digested in the large intestine, and lactose serves as a fermentable substrate for the bacterial flora it increases water flow by osmosis into the lumen. Quantitatively, how much undigested lactose causes these symptoms depends on how much lactose was initially ingested. Also it depends on individual sensitivity, the rate of gastric emptying, gastrointestinal transit time, and the pattern of the flora in the large intestine. This is what exactly happens after the application of antibiotics and diarrhea is prevented. Lactose maldigestion is different from lactose intolerance.

In the Lactose-intolerant people it has been found that certain amount of lactose could be tolerated without any adverse symptoms. Most of these people tolerate >9-12 g (equivalent to 200 mL or 1 glass of milk).

Lactose is converted into lactic acid by lactic acid bacteria. Consumption of certain active strains may help lactose intolerant individuals to tolerate more lactose than they would have otherwise (Lerebours, 1989).

Due to the high viscosity and lower pH of fermented milk products there is a delay in gastric emptying relative to milk which increases the energy yield (relative to that of pure lactose solutions). It is also found the transit time in the orocecal gets prolonged which may be due to the probiotic microorganisms, their metabolic products, or a lower osmotic load resulting from the improved lactose digestion in the upper small intestine. According to Vesa *et al.*, 1997 gastric emptying ($P < 0.01$), and also oro cecal transit time (NS) was delayed reducing the hydrogen exhalation when the patients were shifted from a low- to a high-energy diet. No significant effect was detected on the symptoms of lactose intolerance. Savaiano *et al.* (2011) found that on consumption of native and pasteurized yogurt the gastric emptying was faster. The gastrocecal transit time was found to be prolonged in yogurt as such than heated yogurt (Sanders, 2000).

Several lines of evidence show that the appropriate strains of lactic acid bacteria, such as *S. thermophilus*, *L. bulgaricus* and other *Lactobacilli* in fermented milk products, can alleviate symptoms of lactose intolerance by providing bacterial lactase to the intestine and stomach. Because lactose intolerance affects almost 70% of the population worldwide, consumption of the probiotic products is a good way in dairy products so that even their accompanying nutrients may impart beneficial effects into the diets of lactose intolerant individuals. Lin (1995) and Lin *et al.* (1991) have studied the effect of fermented dairy products on lactose digestion in humans.

4a.8 Inflammatory Bowel Disease (IBD)

IBD is a collective term to describe crohn's disease (CD), ulcerative colitis (UC) and non specific colitis (Scholmerich, 2007). In all these diseases GIT gets inflammated (Damaskos and Kolios, 2008; Steed *et al.*, 2008).

A combination of Balsalazide and VSL #3 (*Bifidobacteria* + *Lactobacillus* + *Streptococcuss alivarius*) was found to prevent such infections (Tursi, 2004).

In the intestine of IL-10 knock out mice with colitis and in humans with Uc the activity of mucosal alkaline sphingomyelinase is reduced. Giuliana *et al.* (2015) have looked into the mediation of inflammation on human cell lines. Yoon *et al.* (2014) have studied the effect of multi species probiotics and their role in IBD.

4b Non- Intestinal Disorders

Lactobacilli and *Bifidobacteria* are usually considered as safe.In the gastrointestinal tract it is *Bifidobacteria* which colonize initially in the new borns and are then transferred from the mother to the child (Borriello *et al.*, 2003). For the dairy products *Lactobacilli* are considered to be good starter cultures. It is rare that they cause septicemia, bacteremia and endocarditis (Cannon *et al.*, 2005). Increased use of *L. rhamnosus* GG has not led to higher bacteremia (Pletincx *et al.*, 1995). Czerucka *et al.* (2007) have written a review on the use of yeasts as therapeutic agents.

The safety of *S. boulardii* is not very clear as *Saccharomyces* is considered as an emerging fungal pathogen. Many times *S. boulardii* has been a cause of fungemia (Perapoch *et al.*, 2000).

4b.1 Allergy, Immunity, Eczema, Urinary tract Infection, Bacterial vaginosis, Arthritis

Allergy

Diseases like atopic eczema, allergic rhinitis, asthma represent chronic disorder.

Twenty percent of the world population suffers from such diseases (Noverr and Huffnagle, 2004).

Many probiotics and microbial products have been indicated to be potentially useful in allergy prevention and therapy by targeting the toll like receptor network (Feleszko *et al.*, 2007). The composition of *Bifidobacteria* in allergic infants has been reported to be more adult like with more *B.adolescentis*. It was found that in healthy infants more *B. bifidum*, *B. infantis* and *B. breve* were found. Kalliomaki and Isolauri (2004) studied the down regulation of the allergic response by using probiotics.

Clinical trials for allergy were treated with *Lb. rhamnosus* GG which reduced atopic eczema during breast feeding (Kalliomaki *et al.*, 2007). The probiotic bacteria increased the immune protective potential of breast milk after treatment with Lb. GG. It was also observed that the lactulose to mannitol ratio was lower as compared to the control. This shows stabilization of the intestinal barrier function. Heat inactivated organism was not found effective. Attempting allergy prevention by probiotic administration has been most successful when assessing atopic eczema, the most prevalent allergic disease at an early age. More than half of the published studies demonstrate a decrease in eczema prevalence until 2 years, whereas the remaining studies fail to show an effect. Effects have been most consistent with combined prenatal and direct postnatal supplementation of the infant and appear strain-specific, with *Lactobacillus rhamnosus* most often showing an effect. Prenatal-only and postnatal-only studies often fail to show effects. Recent long-time follow-ups have shown promising but not consistent results. A very recent follow-up of a large well conducted cohort shows that long-term effects of eczema prevention persists until age 4 and prevention of respiratory allergies might also be possible (Kuitunen, 2013). Prevention of eczema with probiotics seem to work until age 2 years and extended effects until 4 years have been shown in high-risk for allergy cohorts. Effects are strain-specific, with *L. rhamnosus*. Prevention of eczema with probiotics seem to work until age 2 years and extended effects until 4 years have been shown in high-risk for allergy cohorts. These were the most consistent effects especially when combining pre and postnatal administration.

It has been seen that with reduced family size, improved hygiene, vaccinations, use of antimicrobial medications, and the consumption of near sterile food have all decreased or altered our exposure to microbes. Kuitunen *et al.* (2009) explained that probiotics could prevent IgE-associated allergy. Khani *et al.* (2012) have suggested probiotics as an alternative strategy for the prevention and treatment of human diseases. The review targets specifically on inflammation and allergies.

The role of probiotics in allergic disorders

The interest in probiotic therapeutic potential in allergic disorders started as they could reduce inflammatory cytokines and was able to improve intestinal permeability as observed in *in vitro* experiments. Such effects would be desirable in treating allergic disorders. Many studies are underwayto know the efficacy in eczema, allergic rhinitis, asthma and food allergies. Boyle *et al.* (2008) havestudied the probiotics for treating eczema.

a) Role of probiotics in atopic dermatitis

Many human studies and *in vitro* studies in animals suggest a beneficial effect of probiotics in allergic diseases especially in atopic dermatitis has been extensively studied. Kukkonen *et al.* (2008) have discussed the long-term safety and impact on infection rates of postnatal probiotic and prebiotic (synbiotic) treatment: randomized, double-blind, placebo-controlled trial. Isolauri *et al.* (2008) have explained the use of probiotics in allergic disorders especially for nutrition, allergies, mucosal immunity and improving intestinal microbiota.

1. Prevention of atopic dermatitis

In order to prevent allergic diseases the allergens are to be removed. The role of consumption of fermented dairy products and allergy has been investigated and was correlated with the serum levels of total IgE values. A significant reduction in allergy was found among the students consuming fermented milk (Arerugi. 2006).

The effect of probiotics to prevent atopic dermatitis was studied using *Lactobacillus* GG or placebo on pregnant mothers with a strong family history of eczema, allergic rhinitis or asthma also given to their infants for the first six months after delivery. The frequency of developing atopic dermatitis in the offspring was significantly reduced. Probiotics, especially *L. rhamnosus* GG, seem to be effective for the prevention of AD (Betsi *et al.*, 2008). Similar studies have yielded comparable results. The uses of the probiotic in infancy induce protective immune profiles that are characteristic for chronic low-grade inflammation (Marschan *et al.*, 2008). Other studies could relate probiotic benefits to a certain subset of dermatitis patients. The dermatitis which is associated to IgE, rather than other types of atopic dermatitis, was found to come down after the oral consumption of probiotics, namely *L. reuteri* or a mixture of four probiotic bacteria and prebiotics. Probiotic supplementation decreased mean allergen-induced production of several cytokines at several time periods, particularly IL-5 and IL-10 (Peera and Versalovic, 2013). However, Taylor *et al.* (2007) could not confirm such effects in a randomized placebo-controlled double-blind study. The type of probiotic product was different as well as the timing of the introduction of the probiotic. According to Yi-Qi Du *et al.* (2012) this novel approach has stemmed from numerous data reporting the pleiotropic effects of probiotics that include immunomodulation, restoration of intestinal dysbiosis as well as maintaining epithelial barrier integrity.

Giovannini *et al.* (2007) have studied long-term consumption of fermented milk containing *Lactobacillus casei* in pre-school children with allergic asthma and/or rhinitis which gave beneficial effects. Daily supplements containing the probiotic *Lactobacillus rhamnosus* HN001 strain may reduce the incidence of eczema and skin sensitivity in children, according to data from a double-blind randomized placebo-controlled trial the effect of probiotics was not found to be very prominent to prevent eczema. Further clinical studies need to be done in this regard (Daniells, 2013).

Once allergic diseases develop, it is important to control the patient's clinical symptoms. Probiotics may help to decrease the severity of atopic dermatitis and food allergy. Most clinical studies have targeted pediatric patients.

Probiotics in treatment of allergies

Ouwehand (2007) wrote about the allergic treatment by probiotics. Fabio *et al.* (2012) have analyzed data from the randomized controlled studies and evaluated in the review. They have observed that a mixture of probiotic strains is more efficacious than single strain studies.

Gruber *et al.* (2007) did a randomized, placebo-controlled trial of *Lactobacillus rhamnosus* GG as treatment of atopic dermatitis in infancy. A difference was noted between live and heat inactivated usage of probiotics. Folster *et al.* (2006) conducted a randomized controlled trial using *Lactobacillus rhamnosus* in infants with moderate to severe atopic dermatitis and found improvement.

Kukkonen *et al.* (2006) studied the effect of probiotics on vaccine antibody responses in infancy which was a randomized placebo-controlled, double-blind trial and found that it helps in improving allergy.

Prescott *et al.* (2005) conducted a clinical trial to study the effect of probiotics and their association in increasing interferon-gamma responses in very young children with atopic dermatitis. They found that probiotics were helpful and increased interferon yields.

Veckman *et al.* (2003) studied the beneficial effect of *Lactobacilli* and streptococci for inducing inflammatory chemokine production in human macrophages that can stimulate Th1 cell chemotaxis. Perrin *et al.* (2014) compared two oral probiotic preparations in a randomized cross over and found beneficial effect of *Lactobacillus paracasei* NCC 2461 in patients with allergic rhinitis. Suto *et al.* (1999) had used a mouse model to experiment for atopic dermatitis.

Lee *et al.* (2008) did a study in young children on the meta-analysis by conducting clinical trials feeding them with probiotics and found that pediatric atopic dermatitis could be treated and prevented to a large extent.

Weston *et al.* (2005) published their study in 53 infants with atopic dermatitis using *Lactobacillus fermentum* VRI-003 PCC for 8 weeks. After 16 weeks it was seen that the probiotic group had significant reduction of SCORAD scores ($p = 0.03$) while the placebo group did not ($p = 0.83$). Change in SCORAD scores from baseline in the probiotic group was significant but the difference between the probiotic and placebo group did not quite reach statistical significance ($p = 0.06$) evenby the 16th week.

Passeron and Lacour (2006) observed that children receiving placebo treatment in many studies significantly improved in much shorter than expected time. For the prebiotic effect cellulose and maltose dextran were used as placebo, where improvement was seen in the placebo group. The same scientists further compared the effects of prebiotics and probiotics (synbiotics) versus prebiotics alone and concluded that both groups had a significant reduction in the SCORAD scores after 3 months (Van der Aa *et al.*, 2010). Rosenfeldt *et al.* (2003) showed an improvement in children with atopic dermatitis when fed with probiotic *Lactobacillus strains*.

Gore *et al.* (2012) were able to show the treatment and secondary prevention effects by using probiotics *Lactobacillus paracasei* or *Bifidobacterium lactis* on early infant eczema by conducting a randomized controlled trial. They had a follow-up study until age 3 years.

Sonia (2009) has studied the effect of probiotic consumption on sensitization to several allergens (e.g. peanut, hen's egg, soy, wheat, milk, cat, dog), as determined by specific IgE production or skin prick test reaction (SPT). Exact etiology is not clear and the evidence is mounting to incriminate environmental factors and an aberrant gut microbiota with a shift of the Th1/Th2 balance towards a Th2 response. Probiotics have been shown to modulate the immune system back to a Th1 response. Several *in vitro* studies suggest a role of probiotics in treating allergic disorders. Human trials demonstrate a limited benefit for the use of probiotics in atopic dermatitis in a preventive as well as a therapeutic capacity. Vanitha and Agrawal (2012) have purified a protein from probiotic *Leuconostoc mesenteroides* which is active against *V. cholerae*. Agrawal and Dharmesh (2012) have isolated an antishigella protein from *Pediococcus pentosaceous* MTCC 5151 showing that these lactic acid bacteria produce proteins which can inhibit pathogenic microorganisms. Lee *et al.* (2008) have conducted a clinical trial of probiotics on the prevention of atopic dermatitis. Meneghin *et al.* (2012) have given a good survey on atopic dermatitis in children. Michail (2009) has discussed the role of probiotics in allergic diseases.

The role of probiotics in Asthma

Few studies have been done to address the efficacy of probiotic supplementation in the treatment or prevention of asthma. Such studies have heavily focused on the treatment rather than prevention of asthma. Perhaps the largest and the most recent trial were conducted by Giovannini *et al.* (2007) using fermented milk containing *Lactobacillus casei* and studying its effect on asthma and allergic rhinitis.

Between the age group of two and five years of age one hundred and eighty seven children were taken for a study. At the end of the twelve-month trial period the scientists did not find any statistical difference between intervention and control groups of asthmatic children. However, the number of rhinitis episodes was lower in the probiotic group leading the workers to infer that *Lactobacillus casei* might benefit children with allergic rhinitis but not asthmatic children.

One randomized placebo-controlled crossover study examined the effect of heat killed *L. paracasei* on asthma cases (Peng and Hsu, 2005). The efficacy of probiotics in asthma as a preventive measure needs indepth studies to be done and evaluated.

The role of probiotics in Allergic Rhinitis

Role of probiotics efficacy in treating allergic rhinitis are very confusing. Some of the studies suggest efficacy such as the study by Wen *et al*. (2014) evaluated the effect of *Lactobacillus paracasei* (HF. A00232) in Children (6-13 years old) with Perennial Allergic Rhinitis for a period of 12-weeks by conducting a double-blind, randomizedand placebo-controlled study with perennial rhinoconjunctivitis. It was found that the symptoms decreased (Lue *et al.*, 2012). Matsuzaki and Chin (2000) studied the modulating immune responses with probiotic bacteria.

Recently in another study (Giovannini *et al.*, 2007) a randomized prospective double blind controlled trial was done to see the effects of long-term consumption of fermented milk containing *Lactobacillus casei* in pre-school children with allergic asthma and/or rhinitis. Lue *et al.* (2012) checked the addition of *Lactobacillus johnsonii* EM1 to levocetirizine for treatment of perennial allergic rhinitis in children aged 7-12 years and found that it helped the patients. Das *et al.* (2010) have written a good article on probiotics in treatment of allergic rhinitis. Ozdemir (2010) have studied the various effects of different probiotic strains in allergic disorders and have given an update from laboratory as well as clinical data.

With various studies it appears that the use of probiotics may have a potential role in the prevention and treatment of atopic dermatitis, but studies to date have not been conclusive. The unequivocal benefit still remains to be found. However, the effect can be modest and may depend on the target population. The data addressing the effect of probiotics in allergic rhinitis needs detailed studies to be done. Toh *et al.* (2012) have discussed the novel approach of probiotic therapy for inhibiting allergic diseases. Tschudy and Scranton (2013) have shown that the use of *Lb. reuteri* improves allergies in infants.

Immunity

Effects on the immune system

Supplementation of probiotics during pregnancy has shown the potential to improve the fetal immune parameters (Prescott *et al.*, 2008). It has been also seen that immunomodulatory factors improve in breast milk fed infants. Michalkiewicz, *et al.* (2003) studied the immunomodulatory effects of lactic acid bacteria on human peripheral blood mononuclear cells. It has been reported that for patients with irritable bowel syndrome a multi-strain probiotic supplement was found to impart beneficial effects (Williams *et al.*, 2008). It has been proposed that probiotics can be used in association with standard anti *H. pylori* treatment, as they are able to improve patient compliance by reducing antibiotic-related adverse events, thus increasing the number of patients completing the eradication therapy (Franceschi *et al.*, 2007). Many workers have shown varying beneficial roles of probiotic strains (Havenaar and Huisin't Veld, 1992; Lee and Salminen, 1995; Salminen, 1990). These include re-establishment of balanced intestinal microflora, improvement of colonization, resistance and/or prevention of diarrhea, systematic reduction of serum cholesterol, reduction of fecal enzymes and potential mutagens, metabolism of lactose and reduction of lactose intolerance, enhancement of immune system response, improved Ca^{2+} absorption, synthesis of vitamins and pre-digestion of proteins.

Probiotic bacteria help in improving the immune system (Mombelli and Gismondo, 2000). Some *in vitro* and *in vivo* studies have been carried out in mice and in humans. Data indicate that probiotic feeding supported the immune system against some pathogens (Scheinbach, 1998; Dugas *et al.*, 1999) as they produce cytokines, stimulating macrophages and increase secretory IgA concentrations (Scheinbach, 1998, Dugas *et al.*, 1999). Link-Amster *et al.* (1994) examined whether drinking fermented milk which has *Lactobacillus acidophilus* La1 and *Bifidobacteria* could modulate the immune response in humans. They gave volunteers the test fermented milk over a period of three weeks during which attenuated Salmonella typhi Ty21a was administered to mimic an enteropathogenic infection. After three weeks, the specific serum IgA titre rise to *S. typhi* Ty21a in the test group was >4-fold and significantly higher (p=0.04) than in the control group which did not consume fermented foods but received *S. typhi* Ty21a. The total serum IgA increased. LAB which can survive in the gastrointestinal tract and act as an adjuvant to the humoral immune response also (Link- Amster *et al.*, 1994; Ouweh and *et al.*, 1999 a, b). Perdigon *et al.* (1986) fed the mice with *Lactobacilli* or yogurt which stimulated macrophages and increased secretory IgA concentrations (Scheinbach, 1998). With the clinical trials, Halpern *et al.* (1991) fed humans with yogurt per day (450 g) for 4 months and found an increase in the production of γ-interferon. Mattila-Sandholm and Kauppila (1998) showed that *Lactobacillus rhamnosus* GG and *Bifidobacterium lactis* Bb-12 derived extracts suppress lymphocyte proliferation *in vitro*. Food allergy in children caused atopic eczema which was improved by feeding *Lactobacillus rhamnosus* GG and *Bifidobacterium lactis* Bb-12. (Saarela *et al.*, 2000). There is a lot of information on the role of probiotics in immunology (Danfeng *et al.* 2012).

Mucosal immunity

The innate and adaptive immune systems are the two compartment traditionally described as important for the immune response. Macrophages, Neutrophils, Natural killer cells (NK) serum complement represent the main components of the innate system, in charge of the first line of defence against many microorganisms. However, there are many agents that this system is unable to recognize. The adaptive system (B and T cells) provides additional means of defence, while cells of the innate system modulate the beginning and subsequent direction of adaptive immune responses.

Natural killer cells, including gamma/delta T cells, regulate the development of allergic airway disease suggesting that the interleukins play an important role. Intravenous, intraperitoneal and intraplevral injection of *L.caseishirota* into mice significantly increased NK activity of mesenteric node cells but not of peyer's patch cells or of spleen cells. FAO/WHO expert consultation on evaluation of Health and Nutritional properties of probiotics (Chin and Busta, 2000), supporting the concept that some probiotic strains can enhance the innate immune response which include *Lactobacillus* species like *L.acidophilus*, *L.reuteri*, *L.plantarum*, *L.casei*, *L.salivarius*, *L.fermentum*, *L.gasseri*, *L.lactis*, *L.paracasei*, *L.rhamnosus* and *Bifidobacterium* species like *B.bifidum*, *B.lactis*, *B.longum*, *B.breve*, *Streptococcus* species as *S.thermophilus* (Gupta and Garg, 2009).

The beneficial qualities of *Bacillus* spp. were also confirmed. *Bacillus* species (*Bacillus cereus*, *Bacillus clausii*, *Bacillus pumilus*) carried in five commercial probiotic products consisting of bacterial spores were characterized for potential attributes (colonization, immunostimulation and antimicrobial activity) for their probiotic properties. Three *B.cereus* strains were shown to persist in the mouse gastrointestinal tract for up to 18 days post administration, demonstrating that these organisms have some ability to colonize. Spores of one *B.cereus* strain were extremely sensitive to simulated gastric conditions and simulated intestinal fluids. Spores of all strains were immunogenic when they were given orally to mice, but the *B.pumilus* strain was found to generate particularly high anti-spore immunoglobulin G titers. Spores of *B.pumilus* and of a laboratory strain of *B. subtilis* were found to induce the proinflammatory cytokine interleukin-6 in a cultured macrophage cell line, and *in vivo*, spores of *B.pumilus* and *B. subtilis* induced the proinflammatory cytokine tumor necrosis factor alpha and the Th1cytokine gamma interferon. The *B.pumilus* strain and one *B.cereus* strain (*B. cereus* var. *vietnami*) were found to produce a bacteriocin like activity against other *Bacillus* species. The results that provided evidence of colonization, immunostimulation, and antimicrobial activity support the hypothesis that the organisms have a potential probiotic effect. However, the three *B. cereus* strains were also found to produce the Hbl and Nhe enterotoxins and therefore are found to be unsafe for human use.

Products containing endospore members of the genus *Bacillus* (in single doses of up to 10^9 spores/g or 10^9 spores/ml) are used commercially as probiotics. These offer many advantages over the more common *Lactobacillus* products as the shelf life is high and these can be stored indefinitely under desiccation (Ghelardi *et al.*, 2015). Originally, many commercial products were sold as products that carry *Bacillus subtilis spores*, but recent studies have shown that most products are mislabelled and carry other *Bacillus* species, including Bacillusclausii, *Bacillus pumilus*, and a variety of *Bacillus cereus* strains. Product mislabeling raises a number of concerns about consumer confidence (Vecchi and Drago, 2006), as well as attendant safety issues, since some of the organisms found were strains of *B.cereus*, which is a major cause of gastrointestinal infections (Bottone, 2010). Continued ingestion of large quantities of *Bacillus* sp. spores raises the question of what happens to the spores in the gastrointestinal tract (GIT). While no evidence of colonization has been found, it is possible that a spore can interact with the gut-associated lymphoid tissue (GALT). Recent studies have shown that orally ingested *B.subtilis* spores are immunogenic and can disseminate to the Peyer's patches and mesenteric lymph nodes (MLN) (Duc *et al.* 2004). Additional work has provided compelling evidence that ingested *B. subtilis* spores can germinate in the small intestine. This conclusion is based on three findings. First, when mice are given an oral inoculum, more spores are excreted than are ingested (Duc *et al.*, 2004). Second, vegetatively expressed mRNA is detected in the GIT by reverse transcription (RT)-PCR following administration of spores to mice (Gabriella and Simon, 2002). Finally, systemic immunoglobulin G (IgG) responses are generated against vegetative *B. subtilis* following administration of suspensions carrying only spores to mice (Duc *et al.*, 2004). Together, these studies show that spores may not be transient passengers in the gut or they may still have an intimate interaction with the host cells or microflora that can enhance their potential probiotic effect. The following three basic mechanisms have been proposed for how orally ingested nonindigenous bacteria can have a probiotic effect in a host: (i) immunomodulation (that is, stimulation of the GALT) (e.g., induction of cytokines), (ii) competitive exclusion of gastrointestinal pathogens (e.g. competition for adhesion sites) and (iii) secretion of antimicrobial compounds which suppress the growth of harmful bacteria (Baruzzi *et al.*, 2011). Few studies have demonstrated a direct probiotic effect of *Bacillus* spores, but preliminary studies with poultry have provided evidence that there is competitive exclusion of *Escherichia coli* 078: K80 by *B. subtilis* (Ragionea *et al.*, 2001) and a number of studies have demonstrated that *Vibrio harveyi* in shrimp was suppressed by various *Bacillus* spore formers (Duc *et al.*, 2004). A recent study has described the characterization of an antibiotic produced by the *B. subtilis* strain (*B. subtilis* 3) found in the commercial product Biosporin, which has been shown to inhibit growth of *Helicobacter pylori* (Pinchuk *et al.*, 2001). Canducci (2002) have worked on eradication of *Helicobacter pylori* using probiotics.

At the intestinal and systemic levels the immune system functions are enhanced by lactic acid bacteria. In humans, lactic acid bacteria have been shown to increase the B-lymphocytes or B cells, which recognize foreign matter (De Simone *et al.*, 1993), Phagocytic activity, helping to destroy foreign matter (Schiffrin *et al.*, 1995), IgA, IgG and IgM secreting cells and serum IgA levels, which would increase antibody activity (Kaila *et al.*, 1992), g-interferon levels, which help white blood cells to fight disease (Halpern *et al.*, 1991).

The body defense's works by providing a barrier by the mucus layers of the intestine. The mucosa provides a physical barrier, usually preventing foreign substances from passing through the gut. As well, a large variety of immune cells are found in the gut mucosa. This allows the gut to interact with the immune system. Lactic acid bacteria can stimulate immune activity in the intestinal mucosa (Perdigón *et al.*, 1993). In conditions such as allergy or autobrewery syndrome (abnormal gut fermentation resulting in increased levels of blood ethanol), the permeability of the small intestine can increase, allowing undigested protein molecules to pass through (Joneja, 1997). *Lactobacillus* GG has been shown to reverse gut permeability (Isolauri, 1993b). Hirose *et al.* (2006) have studied the effect on daily intake of heat killed *Lactobacillus plantarum* for improving immunity in healthy adults.

Probiotic bacteria have the ability in treating food allergy. This was demonstrated in a recent experiment with infants known to have eczema due to cow milk allergy (Majamaa, 1997). Infants in the experimental group got hydrolyzed whey formula fortified with LGG, while those in the control group just got whey formula. The skin condition improved significantly of the infants who were given the probiotic LGG compared to the control group. In addition, the experimental group had improved levels of factors associated with the inflammation of the intestine. Burnett *et al.* (2006) have shown that immune defense reduces respiratory fitness.

Urinary Tract Infections

Several *in vitro* studies have revealed probiotic potential in relieving urinary tract infections (Reid, 2001). Results have been found to vary for these studies, and more *in vivo* studies are still required in this area to determine efficacy.

Lactic acid bacteria may reduce candidal vaginal infections. One study has shown that women with recurrent vaginal candidiasis who ate 8 oz. daily of yoghurt containing *L.acidophilus* had fewer occurrences of vaginal candidiasis than during the control period in which they ate no yoghurt (Hilton, 1992). Elmer *et al.* (1996) have worked on LAB as biotherapeutic agents for the treatment and prevention of selected intestinal and vaginal infections.

Urinary tract infections (UTIs) are very common in women than men. These are caused by pathogenic bacteria. It has been observed that more than 50% of women have at least one UTI during their lifetime. For most of these infections, patients are treated with antibiotics. However, it has been observed that among these about 30-40% of UTI's recur within 6 months after the initial episode. When UTI's recur, most of the times it is seen that it is because of the treatments which was used to suppress the pathogenic bacteria but the treatment does not last long. UTIs can also recur if a woman is infected by different bacteria.

Over half of all adult women have been seen to suffer with a UTI Urinary tract infection (UTI). In one third women it seems to recur. Older women have higher risk of developing recurrence. Also women who are post menopausal, incontinent and have cystocoeles also with high post void residual volumes.Chen *et al.* (2013) studied the genomic diversity and fitness of *E. coli* strains recovered from the intestinal and urinary tracts of women with recurrent urinary tract infections.Using prophylactic antibiotics as preventative strategies may result in many side effects, antibiotic resistance and *Clostridium difficile* colitis. Therefore, increasingly alternative strategies are being looked for. A safe and effective non-antimicrobial alternative like probiotics is becoming very common. A recent study showed a protective effect against UTI, particularly in women with recurrent UTIs where (Quintus *et al.*, 2005) it is shown that urinary excretion of arbutin metabolites after oral administration of bearberry leaf extracts was controlled. Intravaginal oestrogens have also been found to reduce the number of UTIs in postmenopausal women with recurrent UTI's presumably by increasing intravaginal *Lactobacillus* counts and decreasing uropathogenic bacteria (Marelli *et al.*, 2004) and ultimately preventing urogenital infections. Reid and Bruce (2006) have discussed the rationale and evidence of the role of probiotics in the prevention of urinary tract infections. Liong (2007) has written a critical review giving information on the potential role of probiotics as antihypertensives, immune modulators, hypocholesterol property and peri menopausal treatments. Reid *et al.* (2001) have discussed the consumption of oral probiotic for improving urogenital infections. Aso *et al.* (1995) have shown the preventive role of *Lactobacillus casei* on bladder cancer.

Bacterial vaginosis

Vaginal tissues in women are prone to yeast infections. Chronic urinary tract bacterial infections create significant problems for millions of women annually. Probiotic helps in restoring healthy flora very emphatically. Recently it has been shown that these types of chronic infections are protected with the help of probiotics. When clinical trials were done scientists have found that bacteria of the genus *Lactobacillus*, particularly, are especially effective for maintaining healthy vaginal microflora when consumed orally daily. Oral administration of probiotics in treating bacterial vaginosis along with standard antibiotic therapy is found effective. This also shifts the vaginal microflora from a pathogen-friendly environment to a pathogen-resistant one. Under a randomized, placebo-controlled trial when 64 healthy women were taken, Canadian researchers showed that two months therapy daily using GR-1/RC-14 oral probiotics shifted the vaginal microflora from one typified potentially pathogenic bacteria and yeast (capable of causing bacterial vaginosis infection or fungal vaginitis) to normal *Lactobacillius* spp. Mastromarino *et al.* (2013) have written a review article on the beneficial effects of Bacterial vaginosis by probiotics. Anukamk *et al.* (2006) have proved the use of probiotics by conducting clinical study by taking two probiotic cultures *Lactobacillus* GR-1 and RC-14 with metronidazole vaginal gel to treat symptomatic bacterial vaginosis separately.Yaw *et al.* (2010) studied the efficacy of vaginal probiotic capsules for recurrent bacterial vaginosis in a double-blind, randomized, placebo-controlled study. All the studies have shown the positive effect of using probiotics and improvement in the disease. Lopez *et al.* (1990) have shown the emerging role of *Lactobacilli* in the control and maintenance of vaginal bacterial microflora. Meneghin *et al.* (2001) have studied the micro ecology of probiotics and vaginosis. Paola *et al.* (2013) have written a good review on the clinical trials with probiotics on bacterial vaginosis.

Arthritis

Probiotic supplementation has both direct and indirect effects. Probiotics exhibit direct effects locally in the GI tract, including modulation of resident bacterial colonies and vitamin production. There are also indirect effects exerted at sites outside the GI tract, including the joints, lungs, and skin. Indirect effects most likely result from an impact on immunity, via changes in inflammatory mediators such as cytokines. Modulation of inflammatory responses may be related to regulating or modulating the immune system both locally in the GI tract. It is speculated that inflammation associated with rheumatoid arthritis may be modulated by the use of probiotics (Marteau *et al.*, 2001). Thirty patients with chronic juvenile arthritis were randomly allocated to receive *Lactobacillus* GG or bovine colostrum for a 2-week period (Malin *et al.*, 1997). Immunological and non-immunological gut defenses were investigated in blood and feces. It has been observed by different researchers that gut defense mechanisms are disturbed in chronic juvenile arthritis and suggested that oral administration of *Lactobacillus* GG has potential to reinforce mucosal barrier mechanisms which helps to improve this disorder. When inflamed, the GI tract becomes permeable and serves as a link between inflammatory diseases of the GI tract and extra inflammatory disorders like arthritis. Modulation or down regulation of the immune system and subsequent reduction in GI permeability results after consumption of probiotics (Yukuchi *et al.*, 1992; Vanderhoof, 2000).

The potential of probiotics to control allergic inflammation at an early age was assessed in a randomized double-blind placebo-controlled study. The results provide the first clinical demonstration of specific probiotic strains modifying the changes related to allergic inflammation. The data further indicate that probiotics may counteract inflammatory responses beyond the intestinal milieu. The combined effects of these probiotic strains will guide infants through the weaning period, when sensitization to newly encountered antigens is initiated (Mack *et al.*, 1999; Vanderhoof, 2000).

How probiotics counteract immune system overactivity is not very clear. However, there is a potential mechanism which is responsible for the desensitization of T lymphocytes, an important component of the immune system, towards pro-inflammatory stimuli (Braat *et al.*, 2004). LAB'S are thought to have several presumably beneficial effects on immune function. They may protect against pathogens by means of competitive inhibition (i.e., by competing for growth) and there is evidence to suggest that they may improve immune function by increasing the number of IgA-producing plasma cells, increasing or improving phagocytosis as well as increasing the proportion of T lymphocytes and Natural Killer cells (Reid *et al.*, 2001; Ouwehand *et al.*, 2002).

Mineral absorption

A number of studies have been done to know the effect of probiotic *Lactobacilli* to improve absorption of trace minerals, particularly involved with diets like phytate content from whole grains, nuts, and legumes (Famularo *et al.*, 2005). A study was conducted on rats which were under stress conditions. The rats were fed with probiotics and it was found that the concentration of harmful bacteria reduced from their intestines as compared to rats which were fed with sterile water alone (Hitti *et al.*, 2006).

Other Infections

Probiotics inhibit pathogens through a blockade of epithelial access (Collado *et al.*, 2005). Production of antimicrobials and also acids were supposed to be the reasons in inhibiting pathogenic bacteria (Collado, 2005). In a study done on adults also showed that the infections were prevented with probiotic treatment. In complicated cases like pancreatitis, abdominal surgery, liver transplantation also probiotics were found to be beneficial (Rayes *et al.*, 2002, 2005; Kotzampassi *et al.*, 2006). However, the use of probiotics in critically ill patients for non-conclusive mesenteric ischemia is still underway and needs to reach to some conclusion.

In preterm infants, LGG was administrated for 7 days which was not found effective either for sepsis or urinary tract infections (Dani *et al.*, 2002).

4b.2 Carcinogenesis, Hypercholesterolemia, Dental caries, Respiratory tract infection, Hypertension, Coronary heart disease, Colon cancer Anticarcinogenic effects of pro and prebiotics

These bacteria are able to increase both specific and non-specific immune responses, which appears to be by activating macrophages, increasing the levels of cytokines, higher activity of natural killer cells and/or increased levels of immunoglobulins (Singh *et al.*, 2011; Kailasapathy, 2013).

Lymphocyte proliferation and IFN-γ were measured by Lee and Bak (2011) and activity of selected probiotic *Lactobacilli* was evaluated on the immune function. It has been observed that the strains of *L. gasseri* and *L. plantarum* induced higher release of interferon-γ cytokines. *L.fermentum* LA12 and *L. plantarum* (CJMA1, CJLP56, CJLP133, CJLP243, BJ53 and CJNR26) are more effective in inducing lymphocyte proliferation than the positive control. These strains have been characterized as beneficial in terms of immune modulation.

Lactobacillus acidophilus LA14 and *Bifidobacterium longum* BL05 strains in Brazilian fresh cheese (Minas Frescal cheese) were continuously fed for 2 weeks to adult Wistar rats. It was found that this probiotic cheese is a more viable alternative for enhancing the immune system and to prevent infections (Lollo *et al.*, 2012).

According to Kotzamanidis *et al.* (2010) *L. reuteri* DC421, *L.rhamnosus* DC429 and *L. plantarum* 2035 strains show regulatory activity of immune responses both in air pouches and intestines that was characterized by stimulation of polymorphonuclear chemotaxis, phagocytic activity, combination of TLR2/TLR4/TLR9 signalling and secretion of a certain cytokine profile. Increase in immunity shows homeostasis and provides the host with a capacity to resist more inflammatory response.

Reducing the risk associated with mutagenicity and carcinogenicity

Recently, a lot of attention is being focused for properties like antigenotoxicity, antimutagenicity and anticarcinogenicity potential as the functional properties of probiotics. This has been proved by *in vitro* studies and animal model studies by significantly reducing cancer effects by probiotics (Kailasapathy, 2013; Serban, 2014). Genotoxic substances which are generated within the body usually induce genetic changes or damage. This leads to mutations and carcinogenesis (Wogan *et al.*, 2004, Ambalam *et al.*, 2011).

Lactate formed by LAB and *Bifidobacterium* helps in generating butyrate (Duncan and Flint, 2013). Butyrate has a role in mucosal functions such as inhibition of inflammation, carcinogenesis, reinforcement of various components of the colonic defense barrier and decreasing oxidative stress. Butyrate is also known to promote satiety (Hamer *et al.*, 2008). *Lactococcus plantarum* and *Bifidobacterium* Bb12 have intrinsic antigenotoxic potential and have protective effects against the early stages of colon cancer (Burns and Rowland, 2004).

L. rhamnosus (Lr 231) strain isolated from human faeces possesses the ability to bind with Acridine Orange (AO), N-methyl-N'-nitro-N-Nitrosoguanidine (MNNG) and 2-amino-3, 8-dimethylimidazo-[4, 5-f]-quinoxaline (MeIQx) but not 4-Nitro-o-Phenylenediamine (NPD).The study shows that there is a variation in binding and antimutagenic activity. Instantaneous binding of AO and MNNG by Lr 231 helps in the rapid removal of mutagens which ultimately prevents the absorption in the intestine. A modification of the spectrum of mutagenic agents was observed by the binding of MNNG and MeIQx by Lr 231 which shows residual dysmutagenesis associated with biotransformation and subsequent detoxification of mutagenic agents. Lr 231 strain, which is a potential probiotic for humans, possesses the ability to bind and detoxify mutagens, which may be useful in formulating fermented foods for removal of potent mutagens (Ambalam *et al.*, 2011).

Cancer is caused due to uncontrolled growth and the spread of abnormally growing cells throughout. Every year ten million cases of cancer are found around the world. By adopting certain lifestyle changes and eating a nutritional balanced diet the risk of different types of cancer can be minimized. Most of the cases are found above the age of 55 years which cover almost 80% of total cases. The most common cancer occurs in lung, colon/ rectum, breast and prostate.Colorectal cancer is related to both genes and environment. Around 100 types of cancers are reported. The risk factors are usually due to the environment that may cause mutations and initiate cancer by mechanisms which may be either genetic or epigenetic in nature (Ferguson, 1999). Recently lot of stress is being given to natural diet. Nutrition may supply products that may counteract the causative factors (Johnson *et al.*, 1994) and this can be recommended on the basis of a wholesome and complete diet including probiotics (Pool-Zabel, 2005).

Colon cancer

Many studies have shown that lactic acid bacteria may help prevent initiation of colon cancer. It has also been demonstrated that lactic acid bacteria slow the growth of experimental cancers, although the results are not long-term. It appears that lactic acid bacteria can reduce the levels of colon enzymes that convert procarcinogens to carcinogens. Specifically, lactic acid bacteria can reduce levels of the enzymes β-glucuronidase, nitroreductase, and azoreductase (Fernandes, 1990). Lactic acid bacteria are known to directly reduce procarcinogens, for example, by taking up nitrites and by reducing the levels of secondary bile salts (Fernandes, 1990).

However, most of the reports show the positive effects only during the time period when the bacteria are consumed (Marteau, 1990). It has also been observed that there are changes in enzyme activity in humans after using probiotics like *L. acidophilus* and *B. bifidum* (Marteau, 1990), and LGG (Goldin and Gorbach, 1984). Animal studies show fewer tumors in those exposed to a carcinogen, in the presence of LGG, compared to the animals exposed to the carcinogen without using probiotic LGG (Goldin *et al.*, 1996). In humans, epidemiological reports show that populations eating fermented dairy products have a decreased risk of colon cancer (Kampman *et al.*, 1994). However, further indepth studies are still needed to establish a clear relationship between the intake of lactic acid bacteria and cancer prevention.

Preventing colon cancer

In laboratory investigations, some strains of LAB (*Lactobacillus bulgaricus*) have demonstrated that the antimutagenic effects are due to their ability to bind with heterocyclic amines, which usually produce carcinogenic substances in cooked meat (Wollowski *et al.*, 2001). Animal studies have demonstrated that some LAB can protect colon cancer in rodents, though human data is limited and conflicting (Brady *et al.*, 2000). Most human trials have found that the strains tested may exert anti-carcinogenic effects by decreasing the activity of an enzyme called β-glucuronidase (Brady *et al.*, 2000). Population consuming more of fermented dairy products was found to have lower rates of colon cancer (Sanders, 2000).

With many studies in literature on the effect of probiotic consumption against cancer seems to be very promising. Animal and *in vitro* studies indicate that probiotic bacteria may reduce colon cancer risk by reducing the incidence and number of tumors. A clinical study showed an increased recurrence-free period in subjects with bladder cancer (Aso and Akazan, 1992). As the results are preliminary it needs further study for specific recommendations on probiotic consumption for preventing cancer in humans.

Coronary heart disease is the most common form of heart disease, which is the leading cause of many deaths of people around the world. According to the latest census, it is the number one cause of death around the world. About 12.6 million Americans suffer from this disease, which often results in heart attack. In India in the past five decades, rates of CHD among the urban populations have risen from four percent to eleven percent. The WHO estimates that 60 percent of the world's cardiac patients are Indians. Studies indicate that South Asians have elevated levels of LDL cholesterol and triglycerides, along with the deficiency in HDL cholesterol (good cholesterol, which helps to clear the fatty build up from blood vessels).

Carcinogenesis in Colorectal cancer

It is due to metabolic and physiologic disturbances in the cells which cause cancer. This is directly or indirectly related to the genetic makeup (Giovannucci, 2007). Generally, all cancers involve the malfunction of genes that control cell growth and division. The process of development of cancer is called carcinogenesis. Mostly it starts when chemicals or radiation damages the DNA (Toft *et al.*, 1999). Most of the times the cell repairs this and makes a correction. But, in cancer cells the damaged DNA is not repaired and it dies by the process of apoptosis. The damaged cancer cell has the ability to multiply and make multiple copies of the cells.

Normal cell growth is controlled by various cell cycle check points and shows a normal growth pattern. These are regulated by various genes and protein machinery. During cancer the genes related to cell growth become mutated. They start division and accumulate in a particular area making lumps called tumor's/neoplasms. The normal tissue may be destroyed forming an abnormal lump that may compress or invade forming a tumor. All tumors may not be malignant.

Probiotics have an anticarcinogenic potential as they have therapeutic and preventive strategies. In present situation much attention is given to interventions through diet alterations, particularly consumption of probiotics or increasing dietary fibre. Probiotics and prebiotics may regulate colorectal cancer by changing the colon pH. This may also alter the gut xenobiotic metabolism, modulating the immune system, demutagenic effect and enhance the antioxidant activity. Goldin and Gorbach (1980) have shown the reduction of colon cancer with the administration of *Lactobacilli* spp. (Goldin *et al.*, 1996). Tavan *et al.* (2002) have worked on the effects of dairy products on heterocyclic aromatic amine-induced rat colon carcinogenesis.

Several studies suggest that the effect of diet on cancer development is indirect by affecting the ability of the host to metabolize procarcinogens to carcinogens which may get activated by microorganisms in the large intestine. The bacterial enzymes produce or enhance mutagens, carcinogens as β-glucuronidase, azoreductase, 7-α- hydroxyl- steroid dehydrogenase, glycocholic acid hydrolase and cholesterol dehydrogenase (Goldin and Gorbach, 1976).

It is well known that the probiotics and prebiotics cannot be digested and may reduce the risk of colon cancer by producing short chain fatty acids like butyric acid. pH in the gut plays a very prominent role as an innate immune barrier. LAB has the potential to produce various free fatty acids, organic acids and other metabolites which reduce the pH in the gut. It has been inferred that due to the reduction of gut/colon pH, the colon cancer gets reduced.

Epidemiological studies point out that if the consumption of saturated fats increases in the diet the occurrence of colon cancer increases. Bacterial enzymes (β-glucoronidase, nitroreductase and azoreductase) convert precarcinogens to active carcinogens in the colon. It is thought that probiotics could reduce the risk of cancer by decreasing the bacterial enzyme activity. According to Scheinbach (1998) and Fooks *et al.* (1999) anti cancer activity may occur due to:

- Carcinogen/precarcinogens being suppressed by either binding, blocking or by removal.
- Enzyme activities that may convert the procarcinogens to carcinogens may suppress the growth of bacteria by changing the intestinal pH which may alter microflora activity and bile solubility.
- Altering colonic transit time to remove fecal mutagens more efficiently.
- Stimulating the immune system.

Both *in vitro* and *in vivo* studies in animals and humans show that probiotics have beneficial effects for suppressing cancer. Oral administration of lactic acid bacteria has also shown to reduce DNA damage caused by chemical carcinogens, in gastric and colonic mucosa in rats. The consumption of *Lactobacilli* by healthy human volunteers has demonstrated the reduction of mutagenicity in urine and feces associated with the ingestion of carcinogens in cooked meat. Epidemiological studies, confirm an association between intake of fermented dairy products and reduction of colorectal cancer. The consumption of a large quantity of dairy products especially fermented foods like yogurt and fermented milk containing *Lactobacillus* or *Bifidobacterium* are related to lower the occurrence of colon cancer (Hirayama and Rafter, 2000; Rafter, 2003). A number of studies have shown that predisposing factors like -increase in enzyme activity that activate carcinogens, increase procarcinogenic chemicals within the colon or alter population of certain bacterial genera and species are altered positively by consumption of certain probiotics (Brady *et al.*, 2000).

Inhibition of Hypercholesterolemia by bacteria

Anti-cholesterolemia

Cholesterol reduction with the use of probiotics has been well studied by many workers. The probiotics are known to bind or incorporate cholesterol directly into the cell membrane or produce bile salt hydrolase (BSH) enzyme which deconjugates the bile salts and breaks down cholesterol (Scheinbach, 1998). A study on the reduction of cholesterol has shown that *Lactobacillus reuteri* CRL 1098 decreased total cholesterol by 38% when it is given to mice for 7 days at the rate of 10^4 cells/day. This dose of *Lactobacillus reuteri* caused a 40% reduction in triglycerides and a 20% increase in the ratio of high density lipoprotein to low density lipoprotein without bacterial translocation of the native microflora into the spleen and liver (Kaur *et al.*, 2002).

Hypocholesterolemic effects

Atherosclerosis affects the cardiovascular system and generates coronary heart disease, which constitutes the major cause of death in many countries. It has been recognized that elevated levels of serum cholesterol is an important risk factor associated with atherosclerosis. Along the time, many allopathic medicines have been developed to lower serum cholesterol to treat hypercholesterolemic patients. In this regard, statins have become very common. However, the undesirable side effects of these compounds were observed and have caused concerns about their long term therapeutic use. For this reason, a number of non-pharmacological approaches (including dietary ones) resulting in serum cholesterol reduction were tested. Present knowledge concerning probiotics and their action has been derived from many years of tradition as the consumption of fermented milk products was very common. The various studies done using probiotics and the data collected on various strains of lactic acid bacteria, has shown their positive and benefit action for the health of human beings without any side effects.

In vitro studies have shown that bacteria can remove cholesterol from culture media (Gilliland *et al.*, 1985). A lot of attention has been given to the cholesterol lowering potential of probiotics in humans (Hepner *et al.*, 1979). Hyperlipidaemic patients who were administered *Lactobacillus sporogenes* experienced a mean 32% reduction in total cholesterol and 35% reduction in LDL cholesterol over a 3-month period (Mohan, 1990). One study in hypercholesterolemic mice showed that administration of low levels of *L. reuteri* for 7 days decreased total cholesterol and triglyceride levels by 38% and 40%, respectively, and increased the high-density lipid: LDL ratio by 20% (Taranto *et al.*, 1998). Other *in vitro* research shows that in the presence of *L. acidophilus* cholesterol can precipitate with free bile salts, especially in an acid environment (Klaver, 1993). Either of the actions may help to lower serum cholesterol in humans. Various studies with fermented milk products that have shown no effect in the reduction of cholesterol levels. There is no good evidence to confirm a cholesterol-lowering effect of fermented milk products as yet. The hypocholesterolemic effects of *Lactobacillus plantarum* 9-41-A and *Lactobacillus fermentum* M1 16 were evaluated on rats fed with a high-cholesterol diet. It has been proved that they have ability to lower serum cholesterol, low-density lipoprotein cholesterol and triglycerides levels whereas both fecal cholesterol and bile acid levels have been found to be significantly higher after the administration of LAB (Ning *et al.*, 2011).

Scientific reports have shown that the native lactic acid bacterium from Taiwan which was isolated from the feces of a newborn infant and was identified as *Lactobacillus paracasei* sub sp. *paracasei* NTU 101. When the fermented products were prepared with this particular strain and studied in human volunteers it proved to be effective in the management of blood cholesterol and pressure, prevention of gastric mucosal lesion development, immunomodulation and alleviation of allergies, anti-osteoporosis and inhibition of the fat tissue accumulation. Taranto *et al.* (1998) have shown evidence in mice on the role of cholesterol reduction by *Lactobacillus reuteri*.

Reduction in blood cholesterol and hyperlipidaemia

Cholesterol is essential for many functions in the human body. It acts as a precursor to certain hormones and vitamins and it is a component of cell membranes and nerve cells. However, elevated levels of total blood cholesterol or other blood lipids are considered risk factors for developing coronary heart disease. Although humans synthesize cholesterol to maintain minimum levels of biological functioning, diet is known also to play a role in serum cholesterol levels, although the extent of influence varies significantly case to case. Lactic acid bacteria have been evaluated for their effect on serum cholesterol levels. Clinical studies on the effect of lowering the cholesterol or low-density lipid (LPL) levels in humans have not been conclusive. There have been some human studies that suggest that blood cholesterol levels can be reduced by consumption of probiotic-containing dairy foods by people with high blood cholesterol, however, generally, the evidence is not very confirmatory. Perhaps any effect is small and difficult to measure. Some strains may demonstrate this effect while others may not. The various studies till now show that probiotic bacteria may have a beneficial effect on blood lipid levels. One study in hypercholesterolemic mice showed that administration of low levels of *L. reuteri* for 7 days decreased total cholesterol and triglyceride levels by 38% and 40%, respectively and increased the high-density lipid: LDL ratio by 20% (Taranto *et al.*, 1998). Hyperlipidemia patients who were administered *Lactobacillus sporogenes* experienced a mean 32% reduction in total cholesterol and 35% reduction in LDL cholesterol over a 3-month period (Mohan 1990). In a well-controlled 8-week clinical trial in overweight subjects, daily consumption of 450 ml of yogurt fermented with *Strep. thermophilus* and *E. faecium* resulted in an 8.4% reduction in LDL and an increase in fibrinogen levels (Agerholm-Larsen *et al.*, 2000). Because *in vitro* studies have shown that bacteria can remove cholesterol from culture media (Gilliland *et al.*, 1985) much attention has been given to the cholesterol-lowering potential of probiotics in humans (Hepner *et al.*, 1979). It is now thought that cholesterol removal from the culture media is a result of precipitation of cholesterol with free bile acids, formed in the media because of the activity of the bacterial enzyme bile salt hydrolase (Parvez *et al.*, 2005). The cholesterol-lowering potential of *L. acidophilus* has been most widely studied. Lin *et al.* (1989) performed two studies, a pilot trial without a placebo and a large placebo-controlled trial. In the pilot trial, 23 subjects received tablets containing 3×10^7 CFU/ml. *L. acidophilus* (ATCC 4962) and *L. bulgaricus* (ATCC 33409) daily for 16 weeks, whereas 15 subjects received no tablets. Fasting blood samples were taken before 7 and 16 weeks after the start of the study. Serum cholesterol in the control group remained stable at 4.9 mmol; serum cholesterol in the experimental group decreased from 5.7 to 5.3 mmol after 7 weeks ($P < 0.05$) and to 5.4 mmol after 16 weeks ($P < 0.05$ compared with baseline and week 7). A second study with a doubleblind, placebo-controlled and crossover design did not show a significant effect of *Lactobacilli* on serum cholesterol (Lin *et al.*, 1989; Lee *et al.*,1999). Serum cholesterol concentration reduced after consumption of yogurt enriched with a specific strain of *L.acidophilus* and FOS (Sanders and Klaenhammer, 2001). Certain strains of

L.acidophilus have the ability to assimilate cholesterol. This was shown by the appearance of cholesterol in the cells during growth which was associated with decrease in the cholesterol concentrations in the growth medium. This uptake of cholesterol occurred only when the culture was growing anaerobically in the presence of bile. The amount of bile required to enable the cultures to remove cholesterol from the growth medium was higher than the levels normally encountered in the intestines (Sjovall, 1959).

A recent report in lipid research clinic program included result from a seven year study indicating that reduction of total plasma can lower the incidence of coronary heart disease. For each 1mmol above the normal cholesterol level, the risk of coronary death was 45% higher. Even a small reduction of serum cholesterol by 1% was found to reduce the risk of coronary heart disease by 23% (Manson *et al.*, 1991). Because of the associated risk of heart diseases, there has been a thrust to lower plasma cholesterol levels by different ways.

Three controlled clinical trials (the lipid research clinics coronary primary prevention trial, the Helsinki heart study and the coronary drug project) have shown that the incidence rate of coronary heart disease can be reduced by drugs that lower total plasma cholesterol.

Studies have proved that probiotic organisms have the ability to reduce serum cholesterol levels. According to FAO, Probiotics are live microorganisms which, when administered in adequate amounts, confer a health benefit to the host. It is found that serum cholesterol levels in man from a tribe of Africa and Maasai warriors decreased after the consumption of large amounts of milk fermented with a wild *Lactobacillus* strain (Mann and Spoerry, 1974).

Cholesterol is an extremely important biological molecule that has roles in membrane structure, synthesis of steroid hormones and synthesis of bile acids.

The synthesis and utilization of cholesterol needs to be tightly regulated in order to prevent over accumulation and abnormal deposition within the body. Of particular importance clinically, is the abnormal deposition of cholesterol rich lipoproteins in coronary arteries. Such deposition leads to atherosclerosis, which is the leading contributory factor in disease of the coronary arteries.

Structure of Cholesterol

Synthesis of cholesterol

Slightly less than half of the cholesterol in the body is derived from de novo biosynthesis. In the liver it accounts for

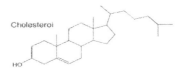

Fig. 1: Structure of cholesterol

approximately 10% and in the intestines approximately 15%, of the amount is produced every day. Cholesterol synthesis occurs in the cytoplasm and microsomes (ER) from the two-carbon acetate group of acetyl-CoA.

The process of cholesterol synthesis has five major steps:
1. Acetyl-CoAs are converted to 3-hydroxy-3-methylglutaryl-CoA (HMG-CoA),
2. HMG-CoA is converted to mevalonate,
3. Mevalonate is converted to the isoprene based molecule,
4. Isopentenyl pyrophosphate (IPP), with the concomitant loss of CO_2, IPP is converted to squalene and
5. then squalene is converted to cholesterol.

Recently, many fermented cereal products have been studied for developing functional food and substrate for the probiotic microorganisms or prebiotics. Cereals have higher content of certain essential vitamins, prebiotic dietary fiber and minerals as compared to milk but have lesser quantities of readily fermentable carbohydrates (Charalampopoulos et al., 2002b). The presence of LAB especially probiotics, in food has been traditionally used as a means of preservation as well as health promoting vehicle (Vasiljevic and Shah, 2007). Phytic acid shows a strong binding capacity for other essential minerals such as calcium, iron, magnesium and zinc. Any such mineral bound to phytic acid becomes insoluble and thus inabsorbable during its passage through the intestines. This characteristic can create deficiencies in essential minerals if no additional sources of minerals are ingested to make up for the loss incurred by the bound phytic acid. Sindhu and Khetarpaul (2003) reported an indigenous mixture of S. boulardii and L. plantarum wherein 24% reduction in polyphenol content was observed. These antinutrients interfere with mineral bioavailability and digestibility of proteins (Serraino et al., 1985) and carbohydrates. Reduction in polyphenol content through fermentation may imply improve digestibility of proteins and carbohydrates and also enhance bioavailability of minerals in the fermented product, thereby improving the nutritive value. There were increased levels of calcium and magnesium and decrease in iron in fermented soymilk as reported by Lopez et al. (2000) in whole wheat flour, where phytic acid was degraded by lactic acid bacteria which led to the increase in Ca^{2+} and Mg^{2+} availability. Kim et al. (2005) reported changes in viscoelastic properties for different dough samples supplemented with probiotic culture which had stronger elastic and viscous properties than control (CW) dough samples. Coronary heart disease (CHD) is one of the major causes of death and disability in industrialized countries. It contributes to (27%) deaths and a crude mortality

227/1,00,000. There is a positive relation between elevated total serum cholesterol levels, mainly reflecting the LDL- cholesterol fraction and the emergence of risk of CHD (Brown and Goldstein, 1984). Reduction in plasma cholesterol levels can lower the incidence of CHD (Levine *et al.*, 1995). Elevated fasting triglyceride levels are associated with CHD (Hokanson and Austin, 1996). According to WHO by 2030 CHD will be the leading causes of death which may affect 23.6 million people around the world (WHO, 2009).

Currently there is a lot of interest in the dietary management of serum cholesterol and triglyceride levels. The current dietary strategy for prevention of CHD is low fat diet (Taylor and Williams, 1998). However, on a long term basis they are difficult to maintain and their efficacy diminishes over time. In recent times newer approaches to reduce cholesterol are being evaluated. These include soluble fibers, soy protein, plant sterols, probiotic bacteria and prebiotic compounds.

The ability of probiotics to act towards the reduction of cholesterol and triglycerides of blood and tissues has been reported in humans (Jaspers *et al.*, 1984) and animals like pigs and broiler chicken (Jin *et al.*, 1998). In other studies by Fukushima and Nakano (1995), also Park *et al.* (2013) the probiotic feed in rat models reduced the total serum cholesterol.

A millet ragi (*Eleusine coracana*) imparts many beneficial effects of which hypolipidemic and antioxidant activities have far reaching health beneficial implications (Hegde *et al.*, 2005). Ragi is valued as it contains important amino acid methionine which is lacking in the diets of millions of people.

Several *in vitro* experiments with *Lactobacilli* (Gilliland *et al.*, 1985; Rasic *et al.*, 1992; Noh *et al.*, 1997) and *Bifidobacteria* (Tahri *et al.*, 1995, 1996) showed evidence for the ability of some strains of these bacteria to assimilate cholesterol in the presence of bile acids. Gilliland *et al.* (1985) in an *in vitro* study found that certain *Lactobacillus acidophilus* strains could remove cholesterol from a growth medium only in the presence of bile and under anaerobic conditions. Because these conditions are expected to occur in the intestine they found out that this should enable the organisms to assimilate at least part of the cholesterol ingested in the diet, thus making it unavailable for absorption into the blood. The purported assimilation of cholesterol by *L. acidophilus* was further supported by the work of Rasic *et al.* (1992). These authors reported that *L. acidophilus* possessed significantly greater cholesterol uptake ability than *Streptococcus thermophilus* and a commercial yoghurt culture. Viability of the ingested bacterial strains in the human gut, and the ability to colonize in the small intestine (where most of the cholesterol absorption would take place), ultimately is expected to be of key importance for this effect. Animal studies have demonstrated the efficacy of a wide range of LAB to be able to lower serum cholesterol levels, presumably by breaking down bile in the gut, thus inhibiting its reabsorption (which enters the blood as cholesterol). Some of the human trials have shown that dairy foods fermented with specific LAB can reduce total and LDL cholesterol levels. Clinical trials with humans are still required (Sanders, 2000). Enas (2005) has written an excellent article on different parameters that can prevent heart diseases among South Asians.

Statistical data for cardiovascular disease

Cardiovascular diseases such as coronary heart disease and stroke are the highest cause of death in the developing countries and are one of the main contributors of disease burden. In India about 70% of coronary heart disease-related deaths occur in people younger than 70 years compared with 22% in the West and 94% stroke deaths occurs in people less than 70 years in contrast to 6% in developed countries. Scott *et al.* (1998) have discussed on the Promotion of Cardiovascular Health in the Developing World.

Second half of the 20th century has witnessed a global spread of a coronary heart disease (CHD) epidemic especially in the developing countries, including India. Framingham heart study (Scott *et al.*, 1998) in USA played a vital role in defining the risk factors for CHD incidence in general population. Major risk factors are sedentary life style, cigarette smoking, hypertension, High LDL cholesterol, low HDL cholesterol and diabetes mellitus. Other factors that influence CHD risk are obesity, family history of premature CHD, insulin resistance, hyper-triglyceridaemia, small dense LDL particles, lipoprotein A, serum homocysteine and abnormalities in several coagulation factors. Multiple studies have clearly shown that CHD is a significant problem in India and coronary risk factors are hypertension, physical inactivity, obesity, truncal obesity and improper diet leads to hypercholesterolemia and hypertirglyceridaemia which are wide spread (Reddy and Yusuf, 1998).

According to world health organization (WHO, 2003) estimates about 16.7 million people around the globe die of cardio vascular disease each year. This is over 29 percent of all deaths globally (www.who.int). Epidemiological transition, with increasing life expectancy and demographic shifts in population, age, profile, combined with life style related increases in the levels of cardiovascular risk factors is accelerating CHD epidemic in India. CHD prevalence in urban population increased from 3.5% in 1960's to 9.5% in 1990's (Reddy, 1998). This rate appears to be higher in South India with highest in Kerala (Enas, 1998; Singh and Sen, 2003).

Control of the cardiovascular diseases will require modification of risk factors that have two characteristics. First, the risk factor must have high attributable risk or high prevalence or both, and secondly, most or all of the risks must be reversible cost-effectively. Blood pressure (BP) is directly associated with risks of several types of cardiovascular diseases, and the association of BP with disease risk are continuous with large proportions of most populations having non-optimal blood pressure values. Fuster *et al.* (2010) have discussed on cardio vascular diseases and health.

Preventive strategy

Smoking is the major risk factor responsible for the CAD epidemic in India. It also causes high blood pressure, high cholesterol and high saturated fat diet. The adverse effects of these factors are very high in Indians. Enas (1998) have recently reviewed it. Better social, economic and cultural status correlates inversely with lifestyle factors of smoking, exercise and abnormal food patterns. Also recommended is psychosomatic modulation by relaxation and yoga. WHO recommends changes in attitudes and behavior (WHO Study Group, 1985). Primordial prevention begins in childhood when health risk behavior begins. Mostly in Indian urban adolescent school children it is seen that there is a high prevalence of obesity, hypertension and hypercholesterolemia due to high fat diet. The need to promote dietary discretion and physically active lifestyle in children is important. A low saturated fat diet and maintenance of ideal body weight and waist circumference should be advocated (Enas, 1998) as a preventive strategy for individuals. When these fail drug therapy is applied. Without risk factors the cholesterol levels should be reduced to <200 mg/100 ml in individuals and in those with CAD or risk factors it should be <160 mg/100 ml. In patients with CAD or vascular disease the LDL level must be <100 mg/100 ml. Naicin can substantially raise HDL and lower the triglycerides levels. Vitamin preparations which contain an adequate-dose of folic acid, B_{12} and B_6 can reduce elevated homocysteine levels (Jha *et al.*, 1995). Consumption of probiotics has shown to inhibit these problems. Kris *et al.* (1998) have discussed in their task force meeting on the primary prevention of coronary heart diseases.

Dental caries

Another very common infectious disease around the world is dental caries. This disease is due to the bacterial fermentation of carbohydrates, destruction of the tissues takes place in the tooth region. The most common caries-promoting bacteria is *Streptococcus mutans* which are acidogenic and aciduric. Probiotics are known to improve gastrointestinal health and inpromotion of oral health. Comelli *et al.* (2002) have selected some dairy bacterial cultures which help in oral health. Scientists are trying to understand the oral disease process and the associated microbiology in the oral cavity. It has been reported earlier that the counts of streptococcus mutans decreases in saliva after use of probiotic containing yoghurts. However the mechanism is not clear. Differences in susceptibility of strains of viridians in Streptococci were studied by Petti (2008). Comelli *et al.* (2002) have discussed on the importance of the selection of dairy bacterial strains as probiotics for oral health. According to Simark-Mattsson *et al.* (2007) it is *Lactobacillus* mediated interference for *Streptococcus mutans* in caries free vs. caries-active subjects.

Acid producers like *Lactobacilli* and *Bifidobacteria* are caries promoting. However many studies have been conducted and they indicate that probiotics have beneficial effects on the caries risk. It has been found that *Lactobacillus rhamnosus* GG (LGG), *Lactobacillus reuteri*, and *Bifidobacterium lactis* BB-12 (BB-12) do not colonize in the oral cavity of adults (Yli- Knuuttila *et al.*, 2006; Caglar *et al.*, 2009; Saxelin *et al.*, 2010). Administration of BB-12 to infants twice a day has shown to have very poor retention in teeth and to the oral mucosa in infants (Taipale *et al.*, 2013). It is not good if the colonization is transient.

Short-term consumption of LGG, *L. reuteri*, and BB-12 does reduce the counts of *S. mutans* (Nase *et al.*, 2001; Stamatova and Meurman, 2009) and the amount of dental plaque also shows a reduction by some probiotics. Dental plaque is associated with periodontal diseases. Consumption of LGG and *L. reuteri* reduced an important virulence factor of plaque (Stecksen *et al.*, 2009). Nahaisi *et al.*, (1986) have studied the effect of long term consumption of a probiotic bacterium *Lactobacillus rhamnosus* in milk on dental carries in children.

Caries in 3-4-years old children was found to reduce with LGG milk (Näse *et al.*, 2001). When Scientists supplemented the milk with *L. rhamnosus* LB21 it was found to reduce fluoride content and reduce dental caries problem in children (Stecksen *et al.*, 2009). Reversal of root caries lesions was found when *L. rhamnosus* LB21 milk was utilized w/wo fluoride (Petersson *et al.*, 2011).

Respiratory Tract infections

Probiotics are known as therapeutic agents in upper respiratory tract infections (URTIs) and otitis where they compete with pathogens for nutrients, space and adherence to the host cells. Probiotics can exert beneficial effects without affecting the metabolism of the host. Beneficial effects of probiotics in the upper respiratory tract infections have been discussed (Popova *et al.*, 2012). The authors have also studied the mechanical actions in the inhibition of pathogenic microorganism.

The reduction in respiratory tract infection and beneficial effects of probiotics has been proved clinically (Reid *et al.*, 2003). Hudault *et al.* (1994) have studied the relationship between intestinal colonization of *Bifidobacterium bifidum* in infants and the presence of exogenous and endogenous growth promoting factors in their stools.

Hypertension

Hypertension has been linked with the activity of angiotensin-I converting enzyme (ACE, EC 3.4.15.1), a key enzyme of the renin-angiotensin system that increases blood pressure. It is a carboxypeptidase enzyme which generates vaso constrictor angiotensin II after the release of C-terminal dipeptide His Leufrom angiotensin. It also inactivates vasodilator bradykinin, giving a hypertensive effect. Due to the inhibition of ACEit is possible to have antihypertension, some peptidesare known for their ability to reduce systolic blood pressure. Interestingly, probiotics have also been reported to exert ACE-inhibiting activity by producing antihypertensive bioactive peptides. Ritter (2011) have shown dual blockage of the renin-angiotensin system with angiotensin converting enzyme (ACE) inhibitors and angiotensin receptor blockers. Depending on the type of dairy products probiotic could potentially generate many different peptides which are strain dependent as studied by Guilian *et al.* (2015). They found recombinant *Lactobacillus plantarum* was an effective treatment for hypertension by expressing angiotensin converting enzyme inhibitory peptide. Probiotics have created a lot of interest, with more advantages to use food-grade microorganisms as carriers of bioactive substances. Probiotics such as lactic acid bacteria have a very complex proteolytic system that comprises an extracellularly located serine proteinase, a transport system specific for di-, tri and oligopeptides, and a multitude of intracellular peptidases. Christophe *et al.* (2015) have shown a surface display of an anti-DEC-205 single chain Fv fragment in *Lactobacillus plantarum* which increases internalization and plasmid transfer to dendritic cells *in vitro* and *in vivo*. Nguyen *et al.* (2015) have shown heterologous expression of a recombinant lactobacillal β-galactosidase in *Lactobacillus plantarum* and the effect of different parameters on the sakacin P-based expression system. During the fermentation of milk ACE-inhibitory peptides were produced which are associated with some fermented milk products in the market. Jauhiainen *et al.* (2005a, b) have shown that fermented milk prepared with *Lactobacillus helveticus* lowers blood pressure in hypertensive subjects in 24-h ambulatory blood pressure measurement. Postmenopausal symptoms may vary among individuals, which is caused due to changes in the hormonal pattern and leads to increased risks of breast cancer and bone health problems. One of the most pronounced changes has been associated with the alterations of pathways in estrogen metabolism. Specific estrogen metabolites have considerable biological activity. Studies in *in vitro* experiment (Swaneck and Fishman, 1988) have shown that 16-hydroxyestrone (16OHE1) binds covalently with the estrogen receptor and leads to long-lasting biological effects. Increased proliferations of transformed and non-transformed mammary cells are linked with increased urine concentrations of 16OHE1 in mice (Lonning *et al.*, 1995). It has been suggested that soy phytoestrogens as isoflavones exert anticarcinogenic effects by altering estrogen metabolism. Kabat *et al.* (1997) studied the urinary estrogen metabolites and breast cancer in a case-control study. The striking inter individual variability in isoflavone bio availability may influence the biological effects on estrogen metabolism. Endogenous β-glucosidase and β-galactosidase activities from selected probiotic microorganisms and their role in isoflavone biotransformation in soymilk have been studied by Otieno and Shah (2007).

Liver disease

Probiotics help in the modulation of intestinal flora and manage chronic liver diseases. It also helps in the hyperdynamic circulatory state of cirrhosis, hepatic encephalopathy, liver function, and nonalcoholic fatty liver disease (Soghra *et al.*, 2012). Sheth *et al.* (2008) have explained about the connection between probiotics and liver diseases.

4b.3 Kidney stones, surgical wound infections and chronic fatigue syndrome.

Kidney Stones

Abratt and Reid (2010) found the Oxalate-degrading bacteria in the human gut as probiotics in the management of kidney stone disease. Massey *et al.* (1993) have discussed the effect of dietary oxalate and calcium on urinary oxalate and risk of formation of calcium oxalate as kidney stones. As human beings do not have the enzyme which is required to metabolize endogenous and dietary oxalate, a toxic compound causes hyperoxaluria and calcium oxalate urolithiasis. Oxalate in humans can be removed via excretion in urine, forming insoluble calcium oxalate and elimination in feces, or oxalate degradation by gastrointestinal (GIT) microorganisms (Marshall *et al.*, 1972). Work has been carried out in *Oxalobacter formigenes* and *Lactobacillus* and *Bifidobacterium* species to study the oxalate degradation which is both species and strain-specific. Catabolic enzymes formyl-CoA transferase (Frc) and oxalyl-CoA decarboxylase (Oxc) are shown in the GIT. The genes encoding these proteins are clustered on the genomes and show strong phylogenetic relationships. Administering *O. formigenes* reduced hyperoxaluria. Similar studies using *Lactobacillus* and *Bifidobacterium* species also show *in vivo* oxalate reduction, which needs to be proved. The ability of the bacteria to survive in the gut is important factor in identifying suitable probiotics for treating kidney stone disease has been explained (Lewanika, *et al.*, 2007) using *Lactobacillus gasseri* Gasser AM63T which degrades oxalate in a multistage continuous culture stimulator of the human colonic microbiota. They have explained the metabolic activity of probiotics and oxalate degradation. Hyperoxaluria is a hereditary disorder and causes stone formation of a special kind in the kidney and urine. Novak *et al.* (2009) studied the sex related prevalence of pediatric kidney stone disease in the United States. Oxalates are naturally-occurring substances found in plants, animals, and in humans. Excretion of oxalates in the urine is a risk factor for kidney stone formation. It is possible that the mild hyperoxaluria be due to over absorption of oxalate from food also probiotics improve gastrointestinal barrier function to decrease oxalate absorption across the gut. In a randomized placebo experiment the subjects were treated for 6 weeks. Patients were maintained on a controlled diet to remove the confounding variable of differing oxalate intake and availability from food (Hoppe *et al.*, 2006). Sidhu *et al.* (1999) showed the direct correlation between hyperoxaluria/oxalate stone disease and the absence of the gastrointestinal tract-dwelling bacterium *Oxalobacter formigenes* which may be preventing stones by gut recolonization or enzyme replacement therapy.

Surgical wound Infections

It has been observed that certain strains of probiotic *Lactobacilli* and their by products may help in the reduction of infection rates in surgical patients and may ameliorate Staphylococcus-related infections of surgical implants. Work is in progress to apply these concepts in the prevention and treatment of wounds and other surgical infections (Gan *et al.*, 2002). They have studied the role of probiotics in surgical wound infections. Howard *et al.* (2004) have studied the current status of probiotics and surgical wound infections.

Chronic Fatigue Syndrome

Chronic fatigue syndrome (CFS) is an illness where aetiology is not known. However, it brings alterations in microbial flora and decreases the levels of *Bifidobacteria* and bacterial overgrowth is seen in the small intestine (SIBO). These CFS patients have increased oxidative stress, have a type 2 helper cell dominate cytokine profile, cause allergies, have essential fatty acid (EFA) status get changed and malabsorption of certain micronutrients. These symptoms were found to be improved with lactic acid bacteria. In addition LAB are strong antioxidants, may improve EFA status, can enhance absorption of micronutrients by protecting the intestinal epithelial barrier, and have been used to treat SIBO.

It is observed that LAB has therapeutic role in this disease (Generoso *et al.*, 2010). Chronic fatigue syndrome: lactic acid bacteria may be of therapeutic value (Logana *et al.*, 2003).

It was found that a probiotic product containing *L.helveticus* R0052 and *Bifidobacterium longum* R0175 improved such symptoms. Oral administration of probiotics may be beneficial and also improves moods. It has been found that it may reduce anxiety. In a clinical trial patients participated in a double blind, placebo controlled randomized experiment with probiotic product for 30 d and found that it was successful in reducing the stress levels (Messaoudi *et al.*, 2011). Candidiasis caused due to *Candida* sp. causes ill health and Chronic fatigue syndrome (CFS) (White and Sherlock, 2005, Truss,1978).Various factors such as immune dysfunction, hormones, poor diet andspecific medications are hypothesized to allow *Candida* to flourish in the gastrointestinal tract. The overgrowth creates many physical and psychological symptoms. Venkat Rao *et al.* (2009) conducted a randomized double blind placebo controlled study by using probiotics to reduce chronic fatigue syndrome. Logan *et al.* (2003) have shown the therapeutic value of lactic acid bacteria in CFS.

4b.4 Lowering blood pressure

Several small clinical trials have indicated that consumption of milk fermented with various strains of LAB may result in modest reductions in blood pressure. It is thought that this is due to the ACE inhibitor-like peptides produced during fermentation (Sanders, 2000).

Probiotics in hospitalized patients

Critically ill hospitalized patients can be divided in two main categories: patients such as multi trauma or severe acute pancreatitis patients who are in an already critically ill state on admission and patients who will undergo major surgery. Considering the subgroup of patients undergoing abdominal surgery, ten randomized controlled trials have been conducted, which show various results, ranging from no significant effects up to 93% reduction in post-operative infection rates. Importantly, no adverse effects of probiotics were demonstrated among these surgical patients. Surgical patients with high risk of bacterial infection, for instance after liver transplantation or pancreatic surgery, benefited most from probiotic administration.

The extent of the critical illness resulting from the operative procedure cannot be predicted, the timing of the induction of the illness is known, giving room for a possibility to start treatment even before the critical illness occurs. Seven studies have been published that enrolled these high risk patients. All three studies that used probiotic treatment pre-operatively were able to significantly reduce post-operative bacterial infections, whereas only two of four trials showed any benefit of post-operative treatment. Moreover, Sugawara et al. (2006) demonstrated that consecutive pre- and post-operative probiotic treatment is more effective in reducing post-operative infectious complications than treatment alone.

Effects of probiotic treatment in 7 randomized controlled trials in surgical patients with a high risk of post operative bacterial infections have been noted.

Safety of probiotics for critically ill patients is most important, as in many cases higher mortality is observed in a probiotic intervention group than a control group in critically ill patients with acute pancreatitis. In one study, 296 patients with severe acute pancreatitis were allocated to receive either a probiotic mixture comprising six strains (four of *Lactobacillus* and two of *Bifidobacterium*) at 10^{10} CFU/day or placebo, starting within 72 hours of onset of symptoms for 28 days. The incidence of infectious complications was comparable between the groups (probiotics vs. placebo, 30% vs. 28%, respectively). However, mortality rates were significantly higher in the probiotic group (16% vs. 6%) as was the incidence of bowel ischemia, which occurred in nine probiotic-treated patients compared to none in the placebo group. Urine analysis demonstrated that in patients whose course of the disease was complicated by multi-organ failure, probiotic treatment resulted in increased levels of intestinal fatty acid binding protein (IFABP), an accurate marker of intestinal mucosal injury resulting from ischemia(Gollin et al., 1993). Furthermore, treatment with probiotics resulted in an overall reduction in bacterial translocation (as gauged by decreased nitric oxide excretion into the urine) compared to placebo-treated patients (Besselink et al., 2008). However sub-group analysis showed that in patients with organ failure bacterial translocation was increased after probiotic treatment, indicating that probiotics had beneficial effects in the moderately ill patients, but deleterious effects in the critically ill. Vander Veen and Abee (2011) have shown that biofilms of *Listeria* and *Lactobacillus* sp. show resistance to benzalkonium chloride and pancreatic acid.

Probiotics and endogenous defense systems

Due to the limited understanding of their mechanisms of action it has become very difficult to assess the place of probiotics in clinical practice, especially their effects in patients suffering from or at risk of critical illness. The available literature suggests that probiotics may have a safer place in preventive applications in hospitalized patients with pre-operative nutritional support than in treatment. In order to achieve success with such an approach, better understanding of probiotic-host interactions both in healthy and critically ill subjects is required.

In cases of severe acute pancreatitis, mucosal barrier dysfunction which are considered critically ill are mostly due to the pathological immune responses which are often aggravated by low intestinal perfusion rates and intestinal oxidative stress. Recent experimental work demonstrated that five days of probiotic pre-treatment before induction of acute pancreatitis stimulated glutathione biosynthesis in the ileum, which results in an acute pancreatitis-induced oxidative mucosal damage and intestinal barrier dysfunction (Lutgendorff *et al*., 2009) continuously when probiotic supplementation was given for five days it was observed to increase gene expression of antioxidative defense enzymes. Increased levels of antioxidative enzymes indicated cellular stress. Administration of probiotics may have caused a minor oxidative assault, such as intracellular accumulation of short-chain fatty acids produced by the bacteria, thereby inducing increased capacity of antioxidant enzymes, preconditioning the mucosa for a major oxidative attack during acute pancreatitis. Initially it appears to be contradictory as compared to the results of the recent placebo-controlled trial by Besselink *et al*. (2008). This shows higher incidences of bowel ischemia after administration of probiotics in the acute phase of severe acute pancreatitis. However, probiotics administered after the onset of acute pancreatitis acts as an extra oxidative burden in an already critically affected redox system (Ammori *et al*., 1999). This causes increased oxidative stress-induced damage and ischemia. When, probiotics are given before an expected oxidative assault it resulted in an enhanced antioxidative ability. This hypothesis is supported by the findings of Sugawara *et al*. (2006). In the study they have shown that only pri-operative administration of probiotics was able to reduce bacterial infections after hepatectomy while post-operative treatment alone did not seem to be effective. It has also been observed that intravenous antioxidant therapy when administered in the early phase of acute pancreatitis showed adverse effects in a recent randomized controlled trial which emphasizes the difficulties of targeting oxidative stress in acute pancreatitis (Siriwardena *et al*., 2007).

With an exaggerated pro-inflammatory immune response multi organ failure is seen in critically illpatients (Clark *et al*., 2009). *In vitro* studies have shown that certain probiotics can activate an anti-inflammatory defense system. Voltan *et al*. (2007) showed that *Lactobacillus crispatus* down regulated the expression of pro-inflammatory genes through production of H_2O_2-induced peroxisome proliferator. Abdel Rahman *et al*. (2012) studied the physiological responses of sheep to diet supplementation with yeast culture. Femke *et al*. (2009) have shown the usefulness of probiotics in acute pancreatitis in rats.

Some serious adverse events with probiotic treatment have been reported as: (a) Immune compromised state (b) impaired intestinal barrier function with multi organ failure and severe acute pancreatitis and (c) central venous catheter. As these factors are involved in critical illness, probiotic treatment is contraindicated for critically ill patients. The Norwegian Scientific Committee for Food Safety evaluated the safety of use of probiotics for hospitalized patients and similarly concluded that probiotics should not be used for critically ill patients, including those with antibiotic-associated diarrhea (AAD), including *Clostridium difficile* infection (Opinion of the Steering Committee of the Norwegian Scientific Committee for Food Safety, 2009, Frøyland *et al*., 2011). Probiotics seem to have a safer application as preventive treatment measures, applied well in advance of the surgical procedure by a propatria study (Besselink *et al*., 2008). Probiotics hold promise to prevent complications in patients at risk of becoming critically ill, especially in patients who need to go for major abdominal surgery. The safety concerns are paramount in this compromised patient group and use in this application is clearly the purview of a probiotic drug, not food. Marteau (2001) has studied in detail about the safety aspects of probiotic products.

4c. Probiotic Lactic Acid Bacteria: Strain improvement

Due to the considerable importance of LAB, culture improvement studies have been accelerated in recent years. Progress in gene technology has allowed this development by introducing new genes to improve bacteria that better fitted to technological processes or enhanced organoleptic properties. It is expected that better understanding of the genetics and physiology of LAB will give rise to better strain use, selection and improvement (Ross *et al*., 2000). Dunne *et al*. (2001) studied the *in vitro* selection criteria for probiotic bacteria of human origin and correlated it with *in vivo* findings. Construction of bacteriophage resistant strains is very important. The resistant mechanisms are often carried out by plasmids and transposons. Due to large number of multiple genes insertional mutagenesis is not practical for protection against low pH. Aswathy *et al*. (2008) used nitrous acid to improve a strain of *L. delbrueckii* NCIM 2025 for lactic acid productivity, acid tolerance and sugar tolerance. Shobharani and Agrawal (2006) have studied the strain improvement pattern by mutagenesis and by optimizing the conditions for culture parameters by response surface methodology for lactose tolerance in a novel native culture isolate *Leuconostoc mesenteroides* sub sp. They found that the activity increased many folds. John and Nampoothiri (2008) studied the strain improvement of *Lactobacillus delbruekii* using nitrous acid mutation for *L. lactic* acid production and found better yields in the mutants.

Exposure of bacteria to DNA damaging agents such as UV light and oxygen or drugs may have deleterious effects on the bacterial cells, particularly on chromosomal structure and replication. Bacteria have evolved diverse enzymatic pathways to remove damaged DNA (Duwat *et al.*, 1992). Little is known about DNA repair in *L. lactis*. It was reported that *L. lactis* has no inducible free repair system for alkylation damage (Auffray *et al.*, 1989).

5
MECHANISM OF ACTION OF LACTIC ACID BACTERIA

The lack of mechanistic understanding of probiotic activity is a major drawback for the prediction of safety of probiotic intervention. The complex gut-associated microbial ecosystem and nutritionally related factors are the most important environmental triggers for the development and modification of chronic degenerative diseases including immune and metabolic pathologies. In fact, the interaction between the gut microbial ecosystem and the host is considered to be a critical factor in overall health or disease. Whether probiotics will exert protective, harmful, immune-stimulating or immune-suppressing effects on a host is dependent on the interaction between the microbial signals, the genetic make-up of the host and the effects by the environment. Many studies have revealed that certain probiotic bacteria stimulate immune cell proliferation and activity as evidenced by the production of cytokines and antibodies, thereby enhancing the effectiveness of the immune response against pathogens. Ng *et al.* (2009) had envisaged the mechanism of action of probiotics. Certain probiotics are able to reduce chronic inflammation and allergy, two diseases that are due to an over reaction of the immune system, by suppressing effector cells and inducing tolerance mechanisms, as was demonstrated for the treatment of inflammatory bowel diseases (Brady *et al.*, 2000; Canducci, 2002). Experimental studies with VSL#3, a probiotic mixture of eight different bacterial strains, showed that this combination of strains directly suppress pro-inflammatory immune mechanisms in an animal model of chronic colitis, in which VSL#3 induced TGF β-bearing regulatory T cells that confer protection to recipient mice after adoptive transfer. These studies suggest that certain strains of probiotics may trigger a protective memory in the adaptive immune compartment (Delcenserie, 2008) that goes beyond their interaction with the epithelial surface. The characterization of specific probiotic structure-function relationships in target populations will limit the risk of inducing converse detrimental effects in the host. Probiotics are generally reported to protect the intestinal barrier, there might be conditions where probiotics not only fail to restore the intestinal barrier but facilitate the translocation or induction of infections. Development of sepsis related to probiotic use in diseased patients has been reported in rare cases (Boyle *et al.*, 2008). The reports about negative probiotic effects clearly show that it is necessary to unravel probiotic mechanisms in the context of the intestinal barrier function and host immune function, keeping in mind that effects are most likely specific for each probiotic strain or mixture used.

The lactic acid bacteria prevent the growth of pathogenic bacteria and help to maintain the micro flora balance in the many ways like antimicrobial activity, decreases the pH of the intestine, releases gut protective metabolites, regulates intestinal motility, enhances mucus production, prevents colonization of pathogens by competitive inhibition, enhances barrier function and immuno modulation.

Important mechanisms of action of LAB are as follows

Colonization of intestinal microflora

A Probiotic microorganism inhibits the growth of pathogens by reducing the pH of the intestine. It inhibits their adherence to intestinal walls, by producing antimicrobial substances such as bacteriocins and defencins.

Production of acetic acid reduces the pH which in turn prevents the growth of harmful bacteria. The probiotic strain *B. breve* has been proved to reduce the growth of shiga toxin producing *E. coli* 0157:h7 by secreting high concentration of acetic acid (Ng, 2008). Ouwehand *et al.* (1999b) have discussed the mechanisms of lactic acid bacteria and established effects of probiotics.

Probiotics are used in many human diseases ranging from GIT related problems to allergies, cancer, AIDS, respiratory and urinary tract infections, aging, fatigue, autism, osteoporosis, obesity and type-2- diabetes. The therapeutic effects of probiotics have been proposed via several mechanisms.

1. Competitive Inhibition: In this the pathogens compete with the probiotic micro-organisms for limited number of receptors present on the surface of the intestinal epithelium. (O'Hara and Shanahan, 2007; Balcazar *et al.*, 2007).

2. They produce antimicrobial compounds like organic acids, free fatty acids, hydrogen peroxide and bacteriocins with antagonistic activity against pathogenic organisms (Gollop *et al.*, 2005) as they reduce the pH in the environment and the pathogenic microorganisms die.

3. With the increase in the induction of mucin secretion the binding of probiotics gets enhanced in the intestinal mucosa. This blocks binding of enteropathogens to epithelial receptors (Schultz and Sartor, 2000; Vesterlund et al., 2007). It has been found that the probiotics adhere to caco-2 cells at the expense of enteropathogens (Pinto et al., 2006).
4. Competition for nutrients in GIT (Scarpellini et al., 2008).
5. It has been found that S. boulardii degraded C. difficile toxin receptors in the rabbit ileum and blocks cholera induced secretion in rat jejunum due to the production of poly amines (Buts et al., 1994, Paton et al., 2006).
6. It has been observed that the immune cells proliferate and the phagocytic activity of macrophages enhances the secretory immunoglobulin A (IgA and IgM) (O'Hara et al., 2007; Rook and Brunet, 2005). They have also been shown to produce interferon gamma (IFN-γ), interleukin 2 (IL-2), IL-12 and IL-18 (Bell, 2007). The IgE production is decreased which gives evidence for allergy prevention (Almeida, 2012).
7. Probiotic cultures are also seen to stabilize barrier of intestinal permeability. Probiotic bacterial Priming of GALT and immunomodulation of GALT response.

Deconjugation of bile acids

The mechanism of the proposed assimilation of cholesterol by *Lactobacillus acidophilus* and *Bifidobacterium bifidum* has been studied well by Klaver and van der Meer (1993). Removal of cholesterol from the culture medium by *L. acidophilus* RP32 and other species was found to be not due to bacterial uptake of cholesterol, but rather could relate to co-precipitation with deconjugated bile salts. Deconjugation of bile acids in the small intestine could result in a greater excretion of bile acids from the intestinal tract, especially as free bile acids are excreted more rapidly than their conjugated forms. Increased excretion of bile acids results in lowered serum concentrations, which in turn decrease the amount of bile acids reaching the liver for secretion back into the intestine through enterohepatic circulation. Deconjugation leads to the reduction of serum cholesterol by increasing the formation of new bile acids. Tahri et al. (1995) studied the assimilation or coprecipitation of cholesterol by *Bifidobacterium* species. Further evidence for cholesterol assimilation by *L.acidophilus* ATCC43121 was given by Noh et al. (1997).

6
INNOVATIVE NEW PROBIOTIC PRODUCTS

Probiotic Fermented food products

An individual requires adequate nutrients like proteins, carbohydrates, vitamins, and minerals to maintain diet. There has been an explosion of the consumer interest in the role of enhancing the health by some specific foods or physiologically active food components, so called functional foods (Hasler, 1998). The concept of functional foods evolved in the year 1990 in Japan.

"Functional foods are the processed foods, containing ingredients that aid specific bodily functions in addition to being nutritious".

Functional foods are obtained from plant or animal

1. Plant sources: oats, grapes, wine, berries *etc*.
2. Animal sources: dairy products, fish, beef, milk *etc*.

Traditional fermented food products play a very predominant role in the diet of African people (Jespersen, 2003). Some serve as main course meals, adjunct of staples, beverages while others are highly prized food condiments (Uzogara and Uzogara, 1990; Odunfa and Oyewole, 1998). Greater part of local staples and many African traditional foods are subjected to fermentation before consumption (Olasupo, 2006). More than 80% of Nigerians consume fermented foods and beverages depending on their ethnic group and local preference (Uzogara and Uzogara, 1990). Traditional fermented foods enjoy wide acceptability among African population due to their organoleptic attributes such as pleasant flavour, aroma and texture, also, improved cooking and processing properties (Holzapfel and Schillinger, 2002). Cereals, legumes, sugary saps and tuber roots are the major raw materials for food fermentation in Africa, but other raw materials such as milk, fish and meat may also be fermented.

Cereals have been the most important food crops in the world (Hammes et al., 2005). In the developing countries, especially in African countries, virtually all the cultivated cereal crops are used for human nutrition and a greater part is subjected to fermentation. The commonly cultivated cereals in Africa include maize (*Zea mays*), pearl millet (*Pennisetum glaucum*), rice (*Oryza sativa*) and sorghum (*Sorghum bicolor*). The volume of cereal-based traditional fermented food products surpass by far that of all other fermented foods such as those made from milk, meat, sugary sap and leguminous seeds (Hammes et al., 2005). Cereal grains are considered to be one of the most important sources of vitamins, minerals and fiber for people all over the world. However, they are deficient in some basic components such as the absence of certain essential amino acids, the presence of antinutrients (phytic acid, tannins and polyphenols) and the coarse nature of the grains (Blandino et al., 2003). Fermentation is the most simple and economical way of improving the nutritional value and sensory properties of cereal grains (Gupta and Abu-Ghannam, 2012). Lactose intolerance, cholesterol content and economic reasons which are major drawbacks related to probiotic dairy products has increased the prospect and popularity of cereals as alternative food matrices for the delivery of probiotics (Gobbetti et al., 2010). Cereals are favored because their products offer the consumers all the three the probiotic, prebiotic and whole grain benefits. Grain based probiotic carriers also resist gastric acids enabling probiotic organisms to be delivered to lower intestine with less loss in viability (Lamsal and Faubion, 2009). Adaptation to high concentrations of bile salts and low pH is important for the survival of lactic acid bacteria in the GIT. The culture *L. lactis* has the ability to adapt high bile salt and tolerance to low pH. The hind gut is the most heavily colonized and metabolically active organ of the body. Colon region harbors around 500 species of bacteria that are involved in fermenting the foods and in releasing bioactive compounds (Conway, 1995). Vidya Laxme, et al. (2014) have shown the synergistic effects of probiotic *Leuconostoc mesenteroides* and *Bacillus subtilis* in ragi (*Eleucine corocana*) malt for antagonistic activity against *Vibrio cholerae* and other beneficial properties. Todorov et al. (2007) reported good growth of *L. lactis* ssp. lactis HV219 in MRS broth with initial pH ranging from 6.0 to 11.0 over the first 10h of incubation, compared to slow growth at pH 3.0 to 5.0. Bacteria belonging to *Lactobacillus* spp. have the capacity to hydrolyze bile salts (Jacobsen et al., 1999; Lee and Salminen,1995). This hydrolyzing activity of the conjugated bile salt protects the bacteria from toxicity.

Food fermentation is a technique which is subordinate to the action of microorganisms or enzymes whereby desirable biochemical changes occur causing significantly modification of food materials (Yadav et al., 2011). Worldwide, especially in Africa, cereal fermentation is mainly lactic and alcoholic fermentation with the predominant microorganisms being lactic acid bacteria and yeasts (Blandino *et al.*, 2003). These microorganisms perform a number of roles which assist the overall improvement of food quality and safety (Olasupo, 2006). Fermented foods are highly treasured for their prolonged shelf life under ambient conditions, their safety and appealing sensory attributes (Jespersen, 2003; Bourdichon *et al.*, 2012). Besides these obvious beneficial effects, other effects are of special importance. These include reduced loss of raw materials, reduced cooking time, reduction in the volume of the material to be transported and elimination of toxic factors (Blandino *et al.*, 2003; Jespersen, 2003). The nutritional quality of food products is also enhanced. The different ways by which fermentation improves the nutritional quality of food products include improving the nutrient density, eliminating antinutritional factors thereby increasing the bioavailability of nutrients and bio-fortification of foods with nutrients (Olasupo, 2006).

Increased awareness of consumer health and the cost of health care, the steady increase in life expectancy and the desire of the elderly to improve the quality of their lives has resulted in the demand and development of food products with specific or versatile health-benefiting properties (Lamsal and Faubion, 2009; Gupta and Abu-Ghannam, 2012).

6.1 The business Environment

Probiotics open up new and innovative potentials to be utilized in medical needs. This creates many opportunities. A very few strains are commercially available and therefore probiotics are not being used as a routine in clinical practice. There have been many barriers in this direction. Many scientists have analyzed as to what are the root causes for this. According to them this seems to be the transition from academics to industries. This also includes regulatory barriers and product barriers (Abenavoli *et al.*, 2008).

Companies preparing Probiotic Products

1. Probiotic curd; Heritage Foods (India) Ltd.
2. "b-Activ" probiotic curd (*L. acidophilus* and *B. lactis*, strain BB12); Mother Dairy
3. "Nesvita" probiotic yoghurt; Nestle
4. Probiotic ice creams, Amul Prolife, Prolite and Amul Sugarfree Amul (Brand of Gujarat Cooperative Milk Marketing Federation Ltd.)
5. Yakult, Probiotic curd with *L. caseistrain* Shirota

6. Yakult; Danone India (YDI) Private Limited
7. Probiotic drugs Ranbaxy; Binifit
8. Probiotic drugs; Dr. Reddy's Laboratories
9. Probiotic drugs; Zydus Cadila
10. Probiotic drugs; Unichem
11. Probiotic drugs; JB Chem
12. Probiotic drugs; Glaxo Smith Kline
13. Fructo-Oligo Saccharides; Probiotic drugs Glenmark Alkem Labs

During the earlier times the primary function of fermenting milk was supposed to extend its shelf life. However, later many advantages like better taste and enhanced digestibility of the milk was found. With this wide variety of fermented products were prepared. Initially the fermentation of milk was done around 10,000 B.C. It is likely that fermentation initially arose spontaneously from indigenous microflora found in milk. Fortunately, the bacteria were *Lactococci* and *Lactobacilli* which typically suppress spoilage and pathogenic organisms effectively. The in-depth study of such products was done from regions of different climates in which they were produced like thermophilic lactic acid fermentation favours the heat of the sub-tropics, mesophilic lactic acid fermentation occurs at cooler temperatures. Today the fermentations are controlled with specific starter cultures and conditions. Some of the many fermented milk products are acidophilus milk, crème fraîche, cultured buttermilk, kefir, koumiss, filmjölk, sour cream, and viili. Yogurt and cheese are also fermented milk products. Fermented milk products can be classified into 3 categories:viscous products, beverage products and carbonated products. The outcome of the product is affected by chemical composition of the milk, additives and starter cultures used. The processing of the product affects the ultimate flavour, texture, and consistency of the final product. Usually stabilizers like pectins and gums are added to avoid the sedimentation of milk solids and the separation of whey in the package, which improves the mouthfeel of the product.

The process, by which fermented milk products are made, starts with clarification, a preliminary treatment of milk followed by fat separation, standardization and evaporation. The next step is de-aeration, homogenization followed by pasteurization. The milk is then cooled to the appropriate fermentation temperature and starter cultures are added.

Starter cultures differ for each product. They consist of microorganisms added to the milk to provide specific characteristics in the finished fermented milk products in a controlled way. The primary function of lactic acid starters is to ferment lactose into lactic acid, but they may also contribute to flavour, aroma and alcohol production, while inhibiting spoilage microorganisms. A single strain of bacteria may be added, or a mixture of several microorganisms may be introduced. The different microorganisms like the bacteria, yeasts and moulds have optimum activity at different temperatures. Thermophilic lactic acid fermentation favors hot temperatures (40-45°C) while mesophilic lactic acid fermentation occurs at medium temperatures (25° and 40°C).

Starter cultures in the milk help in fermentation. Fermentation is the chemical conversion of carbohydrates into alcohols or acids. In fermented milk products both alcohol and lactic acid may be produced, as in kefir and koumiss, or only lactic acidas in sour cream. The bacteria ingest the lactose (milk sugar) and release lactic acid as waste. This results in increasing the acidity. This results in the denaturation of milk proteins and forms masses (curds). This inhibits the growth of other organisms that are not acid tolerant. Following the completion of fermentation, flavorings can be added and the products are packaged, labeled and put into cold storage after which the marketing is done.

Characteristics of fermented milk products from traditional to modern probiotic products

- Kefir is a milk product and traditionally it is fermented by using kefir grains. The grains are like curds and act as a starter culture in the preparation of kefir. Active microorganisms are present in these grains. Kefir grains have a consortium of microorganisms. This mainly contains lactic acid bacteria (83-90%) andrest is yeast (10-17%). Sometimes acetic acid bacteria and mold are also present during fermentation. In the present times however, commercial starter cultures have been developed. These help in efficient product preparation with enhanced shelf life. The microorganism's help in the hydrolysis of lactose. This forms a sour, carbonated beverage which has little alcohol. The consistency is like thin yogurt. The color is white to whitish yellow. The product has a typical yeasty aroma. Although the product is acidic it is refreshing. On analysis it was found to contain compounds including lactic acid, diacetyl, carbon dioxide and ethanol. This also gives a typical aroma and taste to the product as verified on sensory evaluation. There are two Kefir products available commercially. It can be either carbonated or as such when yeast is not added to the starter culture. The product composition and flavor depends on the milk type and on the content of lactic acid in the final product. Milk from cow, goat, and /or sheep is usually utilized for the preparation of the product. Each milk contributes a specific quality nutritionally and sensory.

- Koumiss (koumiss, kumiss, kumis, kymis or kymmyz) this fermented drink is usually prepared from the milk of Horses. It was found to be common by people living in Central Asia. However, people from Mongolia utilized camel's milk for the preparation of Koumiss. The word koumiss is thought to derive from the name of the Turkic Kumyks people. People presume that initially the fermentation would have been in a horse hide bag which contained the microflora from the previous batch. The product is different from Kefir as liquid starter cultures are used. The cultures are *Lactobacilli* and non-lactose-fermenting yeasts. Mare's milk has higher sugar content than cow's and goat's milk, this gives koumiss higher alcohol content than kefir.
- Koumiss is a milky white liquid with a grayish cast and is very light in body compared to most dairy beverages. It is little sour in flavor. The product has compounds as lactic acid, ethyl alcohol. The fizziness is obtained due to carbon dioxide.
- Filmjölk is a common fermented milk product of Sweden. In the Scandinavian countries products like fermented milk have been used since time immemorial which dates back to the Vikings. This product is fermented at lower temperatures by utilizing specifically mesophilic bacteria. Traditionally it was known as surmjölk. Commonly it is consumed during breakfast or lunch. Filmjölk is different from other products as it is fermented using different strains of bacteria, giving it a unique flavour. Filmjölk is a semi-solid product made with standardized fat contents. It can be eaten by a spoon. It Specific aroma is due to the presence of diacetyl and carbon dioxide formed during fermentation in the product.
- Viili in Finland unhomogenized milk is utilized for the preparation of fermented milk. During fermentation a layer of cream is formed on the surface which contains mold and *Geotrichum candidum*. For the preparation of this product starter culture containing *Lacobacillus lactis* subsp. Cremoris are inoculated which creates a ropy texture. Usually it is eaten with a tablespoon so that it can be cut into portions. If it is mixed or eaten with a teaspoon the texture becomes ropy, making it difficult to consume. Viili has a mild acidic flavour and aroma with a thick consistency that maintains its shape without collapsing when placed on a plate.
- Acidophilus milk in this preparation milk with low fat or non fat is utilized. Microbial active cultures of *Lactobacillus acidophilus* are added to the milk. After fermentation the product can be kept in refrigerated conditions. This prevents further growth of the lactic acid bacteria producing sweet acidophilus milk. For curdling it is kept at 38°C. Sometimes *Bifidobacterium bifidumis* also added.

- Cultured Buttermilk this product has been common since time immemorial when the preparation of butter came into existence. Traditionally butter was made by churning milk or cream, but an improved method for fermenting milk became the preferred method for cultured buttermilk production. Cultured buttermilk is pasteurized skim milk fermented by a lactic acid bacteria culture (*Lactobacillus lactis* sub sp. *lactis*, *Lactobacillus lactis* sub sp. *cremoris*, and *Lactobacillus lactis* sub sp *lactis* biovar. *diacetylactis*, and *Leuconostoc mesenteroides* sub sp. *cremoris*) and some other lactic acid bacteria species. It possesses a mild acid flavour with a diacetyl overtone and a smooth texture. Cultured butter milk has a soft white color and may contain added butterflakes, fruit condiments, or flavourings.

- Sour Cream is a product which is very viscous. It is being used since a long time around the world. It is prepared by lactic acid fermentation inoculating *Streptococcus lactis*, with or without the addition of rennet to create a thicker product into cream. For better consistency stabilizers are usually added. Sour cream has a mild, subtle, tangy flavour and aroma which is similar to cultured buttermilk. It has a smooth, thick body. The fat content is around 10-14%. Lower fat varieties are also produced. Sour cream has a limited shelf life due to yeast and mold growth. Giving a heat treatment after fermentation enhances the shelf life.

- Fresh cream is commonly known as Crème fraîche in France. It is mild and slightly acidic in taste. The texture is smooth, rich and thick. It is made in the same manner as sour cream, and used for many of the same applications. Due to the higher fat content (usually 30-40% fat) it can be whisked into whipped cream. It also optimum content of fat and enough protein content to be cooked directly without curdling. (Adapted from Canadian Dairy Commission, 2011).

Utilization of the products in various food products

Kefir and Koumiss are utilized in smoothies, salad dressings, and sauces. They can be added to baked goods such as pancakes, waffles, breads, soups and desserts as a replacement for other milk products such as yogurt or buttermilk. They are very delicious when mixed with fresh fruit or cereal as a breakfast, lunch or snack. They also make refreshing beverages either itself or when mixed with fruits, honey, maple syrup, iced coffees and teas as well as other sweeteners and flavours. Filmjölk is eaten in the same way as yogurt, usually from a bowl using a spoon. It can also be drunk as a thick beverage. Many people add sugar, jam, apple sauce, cinnamon or berries. Cereals, corn flakes or muesli are often added to filmjölk. In northern regions of Sweden, crushed crisp bread is sometimes put into it. It could be used in smoothies, salad dressings and sauces, as well as in baked goods. Cultured Buttermilk is a versatile ingredient in baking. It gives good taste in biscuits, breads, and desserts. Cultured buttermilk is often used in salad dressings and sauces. It is also stirred into mashed potatoes and soups. It is also used to make tangy buttermilk ice cream. It is a refreshing beverage. Sour Cream has many applications. Mostly it is used as a base in dips, salad dressings and sauces. It is eaten as a condiment on potatoes, chilies, smoked salmon and many other foods. Sour cream can be used in soups and works well in baked products like breads, cakes, pies and cookies. Sour cream has significantly less calories than mayonnaise and performs many similar functions. In Russian cuisine, sour cream is common in borscht and other soups. In Mexican cuisine, it is added to tacos, nachos, burritos, taquitos or guacamole giving a nice tangy taste. In Hungary it is used as an ingredient in sauces and in recipes such as ham-filled crepes. Crème Fraîche is sweet in taste. However, the uses are as that of sour cream. Due to the sweeter flavour it very well goes in desserts as a topping, or as a base for other flavours. Crème fraîche works well in dips, dressings and sauces or as an addition to soups. Viili is consumed fresh and chilled, in the same way as yogurt, and can be topped with fruits, nuts, or cereal, as well as other flavorings like spices, sugar and honey. Viili may be added to smoothies, or used in baked goods. It may also be flavored like yogurt. Acidophilus milk is consumed as a beverage and it can also be added to different cereals. It has also been used to make egg nog, sauces and desserts.

Functional Properties of different Fermented milk products

- **Preservation:** Bacteria are inhibited from growing through pH reduction when lactic acid is formed, and shelf life is increased

- **Flavor Enhancement:** The sour characteristic of fermented milk products comes from fermentation products (lactic acid, diacetyl, carbon dioxide, ethanol); these products act as excellent flavour carriers for herbs, spices and other flavorings

- **Texture Enhancement:** Some fermented milk products (sour cream or crème fraîche) can add body and thickness to sauces, dips or vinaigrettes.

- **Reducing Caloric Content:** Many fermented milk products come in low fat or fat free varieties and can be used to substitute for higher fat ingredients.

- **Emulsification:** Milk proteins help stabilize fat emulsions in salad dressings, soups and cakes.

- **Foaming and Whipping:** Crème fraîche is capable of being whipped like whip cream.

- **Nutritional benefits:** Fermented milk products may contain probiotics (bacteria that are beneficial to health) as well as many vitamins and minerals.

Some of the dairy beverage products can be enriched with active ingredients such as omega-3 fatty acids, cholesterol-lowering ingredients and probiotics besides micronutrients. The factors responsible for consumer's inclination towards functional foods are baby health movement, chronic health diseases in aged, changes in food regulations, market opportunities, increased health care costs, changing consumer demands and new opportunities to add value to the existing products with higher profits. Salminen and Tanaka (1995) have written a review on cultured milks and probiotics.

6.2 Probiotic Functional Foods and Reliability

Probiotics are live microorganisms which, when administered in adequate amounts, confer a health benefit on the host (FAO/WHO, 2001). There are several potential and reported health benefits of probiotics when consumed. The major benefit provided by probiotics is maintaining the gastrointestinal microbial balance, which leads to the improvement of gut function (Plessas *et al.*, 2012). They interfere with the ability of pathogens and other non-beneficial microorganisms to colonize and infect the gastrointestinal tract, either by competing for points of attachment in the gastrointestinal tract, competing for nutrients, production of antimicrobial substances or stimulating the immune system (Klaenhammer and Kullen, 1999; Parvez *et al.*, 2006 a,b; Boirivant and Strober, 2007; Singh *et al.*, 2011; Plessas *et al.*, 2012). The improved gut function benefits the host by relieving the effect and promoting recovery from many types of diarrhea, including rotavirus, travellers and antibiotic induced diarrhea, alleviating food allergies such as lactose intolerance and preventing several types of cancer in the colon by inhibiting procarcinogenic enzymatic activities (Boirivant and Strober, 2007; Singh *et al.*, 2011).

In vitro and *in vivo* studies have shown that probiotics could have broader health benefits that include prevention of diabetics, atopic infections, respiratory and cardiovascular diseases (CVDs), improved trophic effect and general wellness of consumers (Boirivant and Strober, 2007; D'Aimmo *et al.*, 2012; Kumar *et al.*, 2012; Plessas *et al.*, 2012; Popova *et al.*, 2012).

There is a growing interest for the use of probiotics with cholesterol-lowering properties in hypercholesterolemic patients (Ramasamy *et al.*, 2012). Hypercholesterolemia, an elevated level of cholesterol in the blood is a well-known major risk factor for cardiovascular diseases, contributing to 45% of the incidence of heart attacks (Kumar *et al.*, 2012). Cardiovascular diseases will remain the leading causes of death by 2030, affecting approximately 23.6 million people around the world (WHO, 2009). Probiotics have shown potentials to reduce serum cholesterol and received attention as a viable option to prevent cardiovascular diseases considering the failure of the current strategies to achieve reduced blood cholesterol on a population basis. Dietary management advocating adherence to low-fat/low-saturated- fat diets appears to be less effective, largely due to poor compliance, attributed to low palatability and acceptability of these diets to consumers (Kumar *et al*., 2012). Pharmacological agents such as statins and bile acid sequestrants that effectively reduce cholesterol levels are however expensive and are known to have severe side effects which include musculoskeletal defects and cognitive impairment (Luo *et al*., 2006; Ramasamy *et al*., 2012).

Various metabolic processes and environmental stresses generates series of oxygen-centered free radicals and other reactive oxygen species (ROS), contributing to the pathology of variety of health problems such as cardiovascular diseases, atherogenesis, neurodegeneration, chronic inflammation, cancer, diabetes, Alzheimer's disease and physiological senescence (Deng *et al*., 2011; Zhang *et al*., 2011; Mishra *et al*., 2012). The ROS are regulated with endogenous antioxidants. The endogenous antioxidant complex is complemented with antioxidant compound from natural (dietary) and synthetic sources. However, synthetic antioxidants can accumulate in the body which can result in liver damage and carcinogenesis but these adverse effects are not reported with antioxidants from natural sources (Deng *et al*., 2011). Several metabolites produced by probiotic strains at the physiological conditions in the gastrointestinal tract have been reported to have antioxidant activity (Zhang *et al*., 2011). This will provide a reliable prospect to naturally improve dietary antioxidants. Probiotic functional foods contain significant levels of biologically active components that provide health benefits beyond basic nutrition. On fermentation, dairy products, meat and fish products, cereal products and many others contain lactic acid bacteria (LAB) that can enhance gastrointestinal function. These bacteria can improve lactose digestion, reduce cholesterol, prevent diaarhoea and can act on the immune system helping the body to resist and fight infection. It is also known to prevent/slow the growth of colon cancer, urogenital infections, alleviating constipation and treating food allergy. Down regulation of the allergic reaction by food has been studied (Kalliomaki *et al*., 2004). They should also have good hydrophobicity which enables them to adhere to the intestinal epithelium and colonize. They are also involved in potential health beneficial roles like immunomodulation, pathogen exclusion, production of antimicrobial substances, anticarcinogenic and cholesterol lowering activities (Ziemer and Gibson, 1998). Fuller and Perdigon (2000) have interlinked probiotics and improvement in immunomodulation.

For LAB to exert a probiotic effect they have to survive the stomach acid (pH 1.5) and high bile acid. They must arrive in the intestine in large quantities and adhere to the intestinal wall. They must also colonize in order to impart the beneficial effect. Finally, the bacteria must show some beneficial effects on human health. These probiotics and its beneficial effects can be utilized by supplementation in various foods (Parvez et al., 2006). The gut flora can be altered to maintain the natural balance and the animal / human would return to better nutrition, growth and health status. These bacteria cause fermentation and coagulation in milk by producing different optical forms of lactic acid (Henneberg, 1904) derived by the reduction of pyruvic acid. *In vitro* methods have been standardized to determine the transit tolerance (Charteris et al., 1998).

These are recognized as gram positive, non-sporing, carbohydrate fermenting lactic acid producers, acid tolerant, non- aerobic, catalase negative and non-motile.

6.3 Is a Probiotic Product Efficacious: Preservation of lactic acid bacteria viability by different methods

Several health benefits are related to the regular consumption of viable probiotic bacteria. Freeze drying and spray drying are well known methods for the preservation of Probiotics. Lactic acid bacteria (LAB) are commonly used as starter cultures for food fermentation. It has been suggested that up to 10^6 colony forming units per ml (CFU/ml) of probiotic bacteria should be present in a fermented food product at the end of its shelf life. To develop culture with longer shelf viability there is a need to incorporate them into food products at the required number. Both freeze drying and spray drying can be used for the manufacture of probiotic powders. Addition of a disaccharide to the cells before drying serves a multiple role by replacing hydrogen bonds lost upon drying with high viscosity thus restricting molecular interactions (Crowe and Crowe, 1988; Crowe et al., 1988; Patist and Zoerb, 2005). Usually freeze drying is used in the preservation of LAB starters but it brings about undesirable side effects such as changes in the physical state of membrane lipids, structure of sensitive proteins and decreasing the cell viability (Lislie et al., 1995). To improve the survival of bacterial cultures cryopreservatives like glucose, lactose, sucrose, sorbitol, trehalose, skim milk and egg yolk have been used (Hubalek, 2003). Panoff et al. (2000) showed that *L. lactis* sp. lactis increased resistance to freezing stress at 10°C. Pre-incubation of *Lactobacillus acidophilus* at 22 °C for 6 h developed cryotolerance during freezing at -80 °C for 24 h (Baati et al., 2000).

Depending on the nature of the compound used, the mechanism of cryoprotective action varies (Saarela *et al.*, 2006). Freeze drying is usually used in the preservation of LAB starters. Studies have been carried out using cryoprotectants (Tamime, 1981; Simione and Brown, 1991). Reconstituted skimmed milk is defined as the most useful suspending medium for frozen or freeze dried starter cultures due to its cryoprotective effect (Simatos *et al.*, 1994; King and Su, 1993). In order to confer the health benefits to the host these bacteria should be viable at high concentrations when reaching the gut. They should survive the stress factors encountered in the gastro-intestinal tract, such as the acidic conditions of the stomach, digestive enzymes and bile salts of the small intestine (Marteau *et al.*, 1993). Shobharani and Agrawal (2010) have shown the enhancement of cell stability and viability of probiotic *Leuconostoc mesenteroides* MTCC 5209 on freeze drying which could be used in food formulation.

Microencapsulation for Preservation of Lactic acid bacteria

An important method for improving the viability of probiotic bacteria in acidic foods is microencapsulation which helps to deliver viable bacteria in GI tract of the host. This may improve the survival of probiotic bacteria in food product or the GI condition (Adhikari *et al.*, 2000; Siuta-Cruce and Goulet, 2001). Protection of cultures by microencapsulation in hydrocolloid beads is very successful as the bacterial cells are trapped within the bead matrix and protect them from the inadequate environment (Picot and Lacroix, 2004).

Developing novel encapsulation systems that would improve the survival of probiotics during processing and storage of functional foods as well as in the GI tract is in need. However, many technological processes and storage conditions are detrimental to the viability of probiotics. Development of probiotic based functional foods holds many challenges (Champagne *et al.*, 1991; Champagne and Gardener, 2005). Encapsulation or immobilization improves the survival rate of the culture (Adhikari *et al.*, 2000; Siuta-Cruce and Goulet, 2001). Among the many techniques available immobilizing living cells in calcium alginate beads were used frequently (Chandramouli *et al.*, 2004). Lee and Heo (2000) studied the survival of *Bifidobacterium longum* when immobilized in calcium alginate beads taken in simulated gastric juices and bile salt solution. Beal *et al.* (2001) have shown that resistance to freezing and frozen storage of *Streptococcus thermophilus* is related to the membrane fatty acid composition.

6.4 Effective Probiotics in the Market Today

A food can be regarded as functional if it affects beneficially one or more functions in the body beyond providing basic nutrition that improves health and wellbeing or reduces the risk of disease. The market of functional foods is growing rapidly the world over. Functional foods are also known as nutraceuticals, designer foods, medicinal foods, therapeutic foods, super foods or even medifoods.

Growing application of probiotic microorganism's that reside in the intestinal tract are frequently associated with health promoting attributes. The market for probiotic foods is growing globally very rapidly. Recently, a lot of research is being carried out to incorporate probiotic microorganisms in non- dairy food products as ice creams, chocolates and juices. Nondairy probiotic foods have become popular in European countries (Stanton *et al.*, 2001). Many companies are utilizing the probiotic cultures in food products (Table3). An overview is well described earlier (Sanders, 1998; 2008).

Probiotic lactic acid bacteria (PLB) in meat products

PLB have been used as starter cultures in the production of fermented sausages (Diebel *et al.*, 1960). Similar roles are contributed for flavours in cured meats which grew over 80% after storage at 20°C for 7 days (Kitchell and Ingram, 1963).

Probiotics in Dairy Foods

Milk is a rich source of nutritive compounds and can be enriched. Milk fat has saturated mono and polyunsaturated fatty acids. Conjugated linoleic acid prevents many diseases. Similarly milk proteins and bioactive peptides protect against many risk factors. Lactose derivatives are utilized to relieve constipation and in the modulation of intestinal flora. Milk minerals are used in the replacement of sodium in salt which prevents hypertension (Shahani and Chandan, 1979).

In developing functional dairy products various groups of experts are needed as scientific researchers, medical experts, nutritionists and microbiologists. Food technologists are needed for product development, process technologists and biotechnologists for processing the compounds, chemists to analyze the compounds and experts for marketing the products. Nutri marketing is needed to explain the results of R&D to health care professionals and to convince them of the benefits of functional foods. O'Grady and Gibson (2007) have discussed the various probiotic products.

Dairy products form the major part of probiotic foods. Milk is natural and forms a highly nutritive part of the balanced diet. The principal carbohydrate in milk is lactose. It is a disaccharide formed from galactose and glucose. It is 54% of the total non- fat milk solids and provides 30% energy of milk. It provides high value protein, vital minerals and vitamins. In earlier days the seasonal variation in milk production led the farms to preserve milk for the cold winter in different forms. Slowly the scaling up was done on bigger scale (Leporanta, 2001). Cultured butter milk and fermented milk products are on the top of dairy foods. Dairy-Based ingredients are used in milk-derived products. Dairy ingredients include fluid milk, milk concentrates, cheese and cheese products, frozen desserts, whey products and lactose, fermented milks, milk fat concentrates. Dairy-Based Ingredients is designed for maximum convenience to the consumers.

To prepare any probiotic milk products it is essential to know the properties of milk, its components, composition, constituents, physical properties like color, flavor, density, specific gravity, surface tension, foaming, viscosity, specific heat, electrical conductivity, freezing point, boiling point and refractivity (FAO/WHO, 2001, 2002a,b). Procedures for basic milk processing, raw milk handling, separation, fat standardization, pasteurization, homogenization, packaging and storage must be known.

Probiotic Fermented Milk

Mesophilic LAB like *Lactococcus lactis* and *Leuconostoc cremoris* strains are fermented at 30°C for 16-20 h (Walstra *et al.*, 2006). Starter cultures other than mesophilic like *Lactobacilli* are also utilized in milk products. Kefir is a traditional fermented milk drink containing *Lactococcus*, *Leuconostoc*, *Lactobacillus*, Acetobacter and yeasts. These also provide a special flavor and aroma. Yogurts are prepared by fermenting with *Streptococcus thermophilus* and *Lactobacillus delbruekii* sub sp. bulgaricus growing in synergy. The fermentation is carried out at 30-43°C for 20h (factors affecting the growth and survival of probiotic in milk (Swidan, 2009). Studies in probiotic fermented milk have been done to check the levels of lipoproteins in plasma (Richelsen *et al.*, 1996).

Talwalkar and Kailasapathy (2004) have written a review article explaining the oxygen toxicity in probiotic yogurts and the survival rate of probiotic bacteria.

The selection of strain is specific to the fermentation time and the flavor of the product. Cheese where whey is separated after milk coagulation is also made by fermenting with different starter cultures. The production processes vary and the products contain live cultures. The production processes vary and the products contain live LAB. All fermented milk products contain live microorganisms unless they are pasteurized after fermentation. The total consumption of fermented milks and yogurt in the EU was 6.35 million tons (Bulletin of the International Federation, 2001). Addition of selected, well documented health effective strains is an easy and natural way of enhancing the functionality of the products.

Dairy probiotic foods can be divided into fermented milk, cheese, ice-cream and added value of functions where the milk composition is changed, functional dairy products with proven health benefits with prebiotic. Texture or the taste of a milk product fermented with a probiotic does not meet the consumer approval therefore it is used together with standard cultures. Probiotics are either added before the fermentations or a little part of the milk is fermented separately and then mixed. Sometimes the probiotic strain is added to the fermented product after fermentation. Commercially, the products yakult (*Lb.casei*; shirota), danone actimel (*Lb. casei* imunitass) butter milk, sweet milk, yogurt, fermented whey based drinks, fermented milks, cheeses, juices and mixture of milk and juice contain *Lactobacillus* species. Milk is a protective food matrix for probiotics and improves the survival of the strain in the intestine. Probiotics are also used in desserts like ice creams. Recently, a yogurt enriched with *Lb.gasseri* was shown to inhibit *Helicobacter pylori* (Fillipo *et al.*, 2001; Wang *et al.*, 2004). Van der Nieuwboer *et al.* (2015) have worked on the improvement of bowel habits of elderly using probiotic fermented milk.

Probiotic fermented dairy beverages

Many drinking type probiotic dairy foods are prepared by adding fruit preparations or fruit essences plus coloring matter (Tamime, 2002). Kailasapathy *et al.* (2008) reported that yogurts containing mango or strawberry reduced the pathogen levels as compared to plain yogurts. Fortification of products with ascorbic acid, amylase or inulin had demonstrated significant growth and higher viability of probiotic cultures (Donkor *et al.*, 2007).

There are many fermented milk beverages in India like chhash, lassi and butter milk. Probiotic drinks in the European market include A-fi 1, actimel. Aktifit, AB-piima, Bella Vita, Bifidus, Biofit, Biola, casilus, Cultura, Emmifit, Everybody, Fit and aktiv, Fundo, gaio, Gefilac, Gefilus, kaiku actif, Onaka, proviva, yakult, yoco activit.

Now in India there is a lot of awareness for better health by probiotic drinks. Yakult Danone India has launched yakult. Nestle India has launched a new low fat Nesvita dahi. Mother dairy has introduced a probiotic curd with dietary fibre b-Active Plusand Nutrifit. Amul has launched probiotic lassi and ice cream. Guerin Danan *et al.* (1998) have studied the effect of yogurt cultures in the fermentation of milk and its influence on intestinal microflora in healthy infants. Guyonnet *et al.* (2007) have studied the effect of fermented milk containing *Bifidobacterium animalis* on the health quality in adults with irritable bowel syndrome on humans.

Successful attempts have been made for carbonated probiotic fermented milk. This was carbonated at a pressure of 15 kg/cm^2 (Shah and Prajapati, 2014). Effect of whey protein concentrate was studied on the survival of *Lb. acidophilus* in lactose hydrolyzed yogurt when kept in refrigerator (Kailaspathy and Supraidi, 1996).

Probiotic Cheeses

Cheese making process consists of lactic acid fermentation of milk a complex biological substrate containing enzymes and varying in its physical and chemical properties. During cheese maturation, break down of the curd due to proteolysis, lipolysis and other enzymic processes gives rise to changes in texture and flavor in the cheese (Kosikowskiand Mistry, 1997).

Cheddar cheese when analysed by GCMS led to the identification of a large variety of compounds as ketones, aldehydes, alcohols, fatty acids and volatile sulphur compounds which contributed to its aroma and flavor. Flavor quality was consistent for a particular starter and any off flavours present were reproducible and characteristic of the starter strain used. The starter culture has a clearly defined role in cheddar flavor development.

Vanaja *et al*. (2011) have studied the volatile profile of compounds with therapeutic importance produced by probiotic culture strain of *Lb. plantarum* LB cfr. and have shown that LAB are helpful for antibacterial activities. Shobharani and Agrawal (2007) have studied the therapeutic importance of volatile compounds produced by *Leuconostoc paramesenteroides*.

Souring of milk is a potent mechanism for the preservation of the growth of pathogens without heating the product. Deshmukh *et al*. (2009) have done a lot of work on the use of chhanna and paneer whey. Whey is an excellent growth medium for lactic acid bacteria to ferment lactose in whey to form lactic acid. It replaces lost organic and inorganic salts to the extracellular fluid and is used to treat various ailments as arthritis, liver complaints and dyspepsia.

Table 3: Companies Utilizing Probiotic culture in food products

L. acidophilus NCFM® Danisco (Madison WI) L. fermentum VRI003 (PCC) Probiomics, Eveleigh, Australia	B. infantis 35264 Procter & Gamble (Mason OH) L. rhamnosus R0011, L.cidophilus R0052 Institute Rosell (Montreal, Canada)
L. acidophilus LA-1, L. paracasei Chr. Hansen (Milwaukee WI)	CRL 431, B. lactis Bb-12 L. casei Shirota, B. breve strain Yakult Yakult (Tokyo, Japan)
L. casei DN114001 DN173 010 (Bifidis regularis™") Dannon (Tarrytown NY)	(L. casei Defensis ™", B. animalis Danone (Paris, France), L. reuteri RC-14™, Chr. Hansens (Milwaukee WI),
L. rhamnosus GR-1™ Urex Biotech (London, Ontario, Canada) and formerly L. acidophilus La-1	L. johnsonii Lj-1 (same as NCC533 Nestlé (Lausanne, Switzerland)
L. plantarum 299V, L. rhamnosus 271 Probi AB (Lund, Sweden)	L. reuteri SD2112 Biogaia (Stockholm, Sweden)
L. rhamnosus GG (LGG") Valio Dairy (Helsinki, Finland)	L. rhamnosus LB21, Essum AB Finland (Umeå,)
Lactococcus lactis L1A L. salivarius UCC118 University College (Cork, Ireland)	B. longum BB536 Morinaga Milk Industry Co., Ltd.
(Zama-City, Japan) L. rhamnosus HN001 (DR20)	B. lactis HN019 (DR10), Danisco (Madison WI)

Adapted from Berg (1996)

Bioactive peptides in fermented milk

The occurrence of various bioactive peptides in fermented milks like yogurt, sour milk and dahi has been reported in many studies. ACE-inhibitory, immunomodulatory and opiod peptides have been found in yogurt and in milk fermented with a probiotic *L. casei* ssp. rhamnosus strain. Also, immune stimulating hexa- peptides have been detected in human casein (Parker *et al.*, 1974). Fermented functional foods with health benefits like Evolus and Calpis available in the market are based on bioactive peptides released by probiotic organisms (Shah, 2007). Lourens-Hattinghand Viljoen (2001) has shown that yogurt is a good carrier of probiotic culture. There have been many clinical studies where consumption of probiotics have shown health improvement like eczema (Kalliomaki *et al.*, 2001; Marteau *et al.*, 2002) and reductions in antibiotic associated diarrhea (Plummer *et al.*, 2004). Fermented functional foods with health benefits like Evolus and Calpis available in the market are based on bioactive peptides released by particular probiotic organisms (Flemming *et al.*, 1973; Table 4, 5).

Table 4: Commercial dairy probiotic cultures and effective colony forming units (cfu/ml)

L. casei shirota	6.5×10^9	L. rhamnosus GG	10^9 þ 10^{10}
L. plantarum 299 v	5.0×10^8	L. acidophilus NCFB 1748	3 þ 10^{11}
L. reuteri	$1.0 \times 10^8\text{-}10^{11}$	L. rhamnosus DSM 6594	16 þ 10^9

Source: Anonymous (2011)

Table 5: Commercial dairy products and ingredients with health or function claims based on bioactive peptides

Brand name	Product	Functional bioactive peptide	Health/ Function claim
Calpis	Sour milk	Val-Pro-pro, Ile-pro-pro from casein and k-casein	Reduction blood pressure
Biozate	Hydrolysed whey protein isolate	β-lactoglobulin fragments	Reduction blood pressure
Product F200/ Lactium	Flavored milk, drink, confectionery, capsule	As 1-casein (91-100) (Try-Leu-Gly-Tyr-Leu-Glu-Gln-Leu-Leu-Arg)	Reduction of stress effects
Capolac	Ingredient	Casein phosphor peptide	Helps mineral absorption

Source: Dziuba and Dziuba, 2014.

Cereal based probiotic fermented dairy beverages

Addition of cereals into milk enriches the mineral value and fibre. Probiotic fermentation enhances the nutritive value, palatability and functionality of cereals. It also reduces antinutritional factors. Millets like sorghum, ragi and jowar are utilized. Cereal solids are incorporated into milk before and after fermentation (Gupta et al., 2007). Charalampopoulos et al. (2002 a) have studied the growth pattern of lactic acid bacteria in cereal substrates.

Cereals offer another alternative for the production of probiotic functional foods. The multiple beneficial effects of cereals can be exploited in different ways leading to the design of novel cereal foods or cereal ingredients that can target specific populations. Cereals can be utilized as substrate for fermentation for the growth of PLB. However, it is important to know the composition and processing of cereal grains, the formulation of the substrate, the growth pattern and viability in the form of colony forming units of the starter culture, stability of the culture during the shelf life, organoleptic and sensory properties and the nutritional value of the final product (Wood, 1997).

Cereals contain water soluble fibre like β-glucan and arabinoxylan, oligosaccharides like gluco and fructo oligosaccharides and resistant starch which act as prebiotics.

The development of non- dairy probiotic product is a challenge to the food industry in its effort to utilize the abundant natural resources by producing high quality functional products. In this regard baby foods and confectionery formulations have been developed with supplementing probiotic culture (Saarela *et al.*, 2000).

Lactic acid fermentation of cereals has been established for a very long time especially being used in Asia and Africa for producing beverages, gruels and porridge. The preparation procedure is usually general by taking grains like maize, sorghum or millet grains which are soaked in clean water for 1-2 days. The grains become soft and are then milled into slurry. Hull, bran are removed after sieving and then fermented. The pH decreases and the acidity increases due to acid production by PLB.

In the west usually wheat and rye are used for sourdough preparation. The population of culture in fully fermented sourdoughs is more than 10^9 cfu/ml. The good growth of PLB in cereals suggests that the incorporation of a human derived prebiotic strain in a cereal substrate under controlled conditions would produce a fermented food with defined and consistent characteristics with health promoting properties. However, it is important to look into many of the technological aspects like composition and processing of the cereal grain and PLB. High cell growth rate and acidification may result in reduction of fermentation times and enhance the viability of the specific strain by preventing the growth of undesirable microorganisms present in the raw material (Marklinder and Lonner, 1992). Adaptability of the probiotic in the substrate is a very important criterion in the selection procedure of a suitable strain (Oberman and Libudzisz, 1998).

The culture strains have very particular nutritional requirements for carbohydrates, amino acids, peptides, fatty esters, salts, nucleic acid derivatives and vitamins (Severson, 1998). Many homo fermentative and hetero fermentative lactic acid bacteria were tested and oats were found to be a suitable substrate for the growth of Probiotic lactic acid bacteria. *Lb. acidophilus* was found to grow slowly. The highest viability was found with *Lb. plantarum* and *Lb. reuteri* (Mills *et al.*, 2011).

Using malt, barley or wheat as media for probiotic culture the malt medium was found best (Charalampopoulos *et al.*, 2002 a, b). It was also found to be strain specific. *Lb. plantarum* had the ability to tolerate low pH by maintaining a proton and charge gradient.

Survival of the probiotic strains during gastric transit is also influenced by the physico chemical properties of the food carrier used for delivery. The buffering capacity and the pH of the carrier medium are significant factors, as food formulations with pH ranging from 3.5 to 4.5 and high buffering capacity will increase the pH of the gastric tract and thus enhance the stability of the probiotic strain (Kailaspathy and Chin, 2000).

The grains of corn, sorghum, millet, barley, rye and oats contain a lot of crude fibre and lack gluten like proteins of wheat. The traditional foods from these grains lack flavor and aroma (Abdel-Haleem, 2008). The fermentation with PLB improves the sensorial value, volatiles as higher alcohols, aldehydes, ethyl acetate and diacetyl are formed (Agrawal *et al.*, 2000). In general a single strain of LAB is not very acceptable and therefore in order to enhance the aromatic profile of the final product many strains are incorporated to bring out the desired flavor. It is important to study the metabolism of all the culture strains so that they grow in the cereal substrate and do not act antagonistically towards each other. Vanaja *et al.* (2011) have shown the formation of volatiles and fatty acids of therapeutic importance in the probiotic *Lactobacillus plantarum* L Pc fr which was adapted to resist GIT conditions.

Cereals are generally suitable substrates for the growth of human derived probiotic strains. A systematic approach is needed in order to identify the intrinsic and processing factors that could enhance the growth and survival of the probiotic strain *in vitro* and *in vivo*. The improvement in the organoleptic properties can be done using supporting cultures that act synergistically on the probiotic strains. The functionality of colonic strains could be improved by the presence of specific non digestible components of the cereal matrix that could act as prebiotic. The possibility of separating specific fractions of non-digestible soluble fibre from different types of cereals or cereal by products through processing technologies as pearling and sieving or enzymatic modifications will be helpful. Steinkraus (1996) has discussed in depth the indigenous fermented foods. Svanberg (1995) has discussed lactic acid fermented foods for feeding infants.

Fermentation of Sauerkraut

New cultivars of cabbage are constantly being developed to confirm the ever changing agricultural and ecological demands. Sauerkraut fermentation is a model system for the study of growth of mixed cultures and their biological control. Environmental factors like substrate composition, anaerobiosis, temperature, pH, salt concentration serve as a means to modify and direct the interactions of a microbial flora. Even in poultry products (La Ragione *et al.* 2001) have shown that *Bacillus subtilis* spores competitively exclude *E.coli* O78:k80.

For the commercial production a controlled fermentation and information on the role and limitations of the undesirable or abnormal end product formation is necessary to establish conditions which are optimal for the growth of selective cultures (Stamer *et al.*, 1971).

Brined cucumbers

The process is favoured by the introduction of starter cultures with the control of undesirable microbial activity. Brining treatments, environmental conditions and initial microbial populations are primary factors which decide the course of microbial activity. Mainly the fermentation is by homofermentative LAB.

Probiotics in production of Soy sauce

Soy sauce and sourdough both utilize the interaction between yeasts and *Lactobacilli* which contribute to the flavor of the final product (Yong and Wood, 1976). In the sourdough bread fermentation lactic acid is produced by the bacterium which contributes to a distinctive flavor and texture of the finished bread. In the sour fermentation there is co-existence of bacteria and yeast. Enhanced growth of *Lactobacilli* on immobilization has been studied in soy milk.

Probiotic Tempeh

Tempeh is a fermented soybean product covered with white mold, a compact cake produced by the fermentation of dehulled, hydrated, soaked and precooked soybean cotyledons. The fermenting organism is *Rhizopus oligosporus*. The fungus improves the flavor and aroma of the product. Tempeh is a traditional fermented food in Indonesia. It is rich in calories, proteins, amino acids, vitamins, minerals, antioxidants, antimicrobials and dietary fibers. Biotechnologically, it is nutritionally rich with nutty taste, odor of fresh mushroom and nougat like texture. It can be consumed from infants to aged people.

Today, it is very common in countries like Malaysia, Holland, Canada and West Indies. The substrates overgrown with desirable, edible microorganisms become resistant to invasion by spoilage, food poisoning and toxin producing microorganisms. It is beneficial for health as it decreases risk of heart diseases, strokes, osteoporosis, cancer, digestive disorders and reduction of fat.

There are other cereals and legume substrates like chick pea, horse gram, lupin, common bean, ground nut, wheat and maize which are used for tempeh preparation. Soya milk has also been utilized for the tempeh production. Tempeh when fresh is perishable due to sporulation by fungi. Therefore, there is a practice to blanch the tempeh product, dry and powder it which can be stored for longer time. However, tempeh contains small amounts of oxalates which if accumulated can cause health problems.

Fermentation of soybean improves digestibility by reduction of antinutritional factors like tannin and phytate in addition to production of acids which inhibit the production of pathogenic bacteria which is important in the manufacture of food. They are low cost nutritious food which can be consumed by all socio economic groups.

For developing new foods large marketing campaigns are required and the consumer needs to adapt to the new product. Developing new and innovative products or reformulations of the ones which are existing enables the manufacturer to meet the expectations of the consumers who are very health conscious today.

Cereals are gaining a lot of importance for preparing probiotic foods as they have the ability to grow and deliver probiotic LAB to the human gut along with prebiotic compounds.

Probiotic fermented foods with specific functions

Steinkraus (1996) defined indigenous fermented foods as foods where microorganisms bring about some biochemical changes in the substances during fermentation and enrichment of the human diet through the development of a flavour, aroma and texture in the foods. The remarkable aspects of fermented foods is that they have biological functions enhancing several health promoting benefits for the consumers due to the functional microorganisms associated with them. Bio enrichment of nutritional value, protective properties, bioavailability of minerals, therapeutic value, production of antioxidants and immunological effects are some of the biological functions of fermented foods (Tamang, 2007). In a recent study, formulated synbiotic tarhana (Turkish fermented cereal food) was produced as a functional food from the fermentation of wheat flour, some spices [salt, pepper, dill and sweet marjoram, some vegetables (tomato), pepper (*Capsicum annum*) and onion, and synbiotic yoghurt which prepared with prebiotic (inulin and lactose each 3%) and different concentrations of the probiotic culture containing *Streptococcus thermophilus*, *Lactobacillus acidophilus* and *Bifidobacterium bifidum*. After fermentation, it was dried. The effect of dried tarhana on the plasma lipid profile of human subjects was studied. Subjects supplemented with dried tarhana showed significant reduction in total plasma cholesterol, low density lipoproteins (LDL-C) and triglycerides, while high density lipoprotein (HDL-C) increased (Gabrial *et al.*, 2010).

A study suggests that LAB strains, such as *L. rhamnosus* BFE5264 and *L. plantarum* NR74, may promote cholesterol efflux in enterocytes, and thus potentially contribute to the prevention of hypercholesterolemia and atherosclerosis (Yoon *et al.*, 2011).

A symbiotic shake was developed and manufactured by the company Maxinutri Alimentos LTDA using specific formulation containing 4.5% fructo-oligosaccharide (Corns Products), 2% *Lactobacillus acidophilus* (Fortitech), 2% *Bifidobacterium bifidum* (Fortitech).The placebo shake was manufactured the same way as the symbiotic dry mix, but without the addition of the probiotics *Lactobacillus acidophilus* and *Bifidobacterium bifidum*, or the prebiotic fructooligosaccharide. The effect of the consumption of the new symbiotic shake on glycemia and cholesterol levels in elderly people with type 2 diabetes mellitus was studied. The results of the symbiotic group showed a non-significant reduction ($P > 0.05$) in total cholesterol and triglycerides, a significant increase ($P < 0.05$) in HDL cholesterol and a significant reduction ($P < 0.05$) in fasting glycemia. No significant changes were observed in the placebo group (Moroti *et al.*, 2012).

Cereal based fermented foods

Cereals are high in starch, dietary fiber, vitamins and minerals, but typical amounts and quality of protein present do not fulfil the nutritional requirements of animals (McDonald *et al.*, 2002). Thus, cereal based feeds are amended with additional protein sources to attain the required protein levels. The addition and proliferation of microorganisms in feed may improve the nutritional quality for the animals.

Wheat (*Triticum aestivum*) is an excellent fodder cereal, with high energy and low bran content, but the protein quality is generally poor (Shewry, 2007). The high starch content also limits the use of wheat in ruminant feeds, as it might perturb the rumen fermentation (McDonald *et al.*, 2002). More specifically, a validation of the protein quality is necessary, as the proportion of essential amino acids often decreases when crude protein content increases (Simonsson, 1995; Shewry, 2007). Abdel Haleem *et al.* (2008) have studied the effect of fermentation on antinutritional factors of sorghum.

Tamang (2010) defined ethnic, fermented foods as foods from locally available raw materials of plant or animal sources either naturally or by adding starter cultures containing functional microorganisms that modify the substrates biochemically and organoleptically into edible products that are culturally and socially acceptable to the consumers.

Functional foods can be defined as any food that may provide a health benefit beyond the traditional nutrients they contain (Williams *et al.*, 2006). Such foods may contain one or a combination of components that have desirable cellular or physiological effects on the body (Champagne and Gardner 2005). During food fermentation, microorganisms have contributed to food functionality through their enzyme portfolio and the release of active metabolites (Gobbetti *et al.*, 2010). Probiotic properties of microorganisms have also contributed to the important roles in conferring functional properties, especially when fermented foods have been reported to reduce the severity, duration and morbidity of diarrhea and confer several other health benefits on consumers (Jespersen, 2003).

Soymilk, the water extract of soybeans (*Glycine max* (L.) Merrill) is a rich source of protein, iron, calcium and unsaturated fatty acids as well as free of lactose that serve as asubstitute for dairy milk, the lactose-intolerant consumers and milk-allergy patients can also consume this product (Yang and Zhang, 2009). The high nutritive value and health characteristics of soymilk encourage the consumers, but due to their beany flavor and indigestible oligosaccharides their popularity is limited (Girigowda and Mulimani, 2006). Recently, fermentation of soy milk is being carried out with various microorganisms, especially lactic acid bacteria (LAB) and *Bifidobacteria* (Chou and Hou, 2000; Beasley *et al.*, 2003). Fermentation of soymilk not only improves the bioavailability of isoflavones, it also removes the undesirable beany flavor, the digestibility of protein increases, providing more soluble calcium. It enhances intestinal health, and supports immune system. In addition, soy-based foods are known to behypolipidemic, anticholesterolemic, antiallergic and antiatherogenic. They also reduce the prevailing proteinmalnutrition problems (Kalaiselvan *et al.*, 2010).

As spore formers, bacilli are more robust and can resist the down stream processing better then LAB and are better survivors under gastrointestinal condition of consumers. They are potential probiotics. *Bacillus* spp. has a longer logarithmic phase giving an advantage to the food industries, ability to produce a variety of extracellular enzymes that are stable at wide range of pH and temperature. *Bacillus subtilis* (natto) is one of the popular starter culture used in production of natto, a traditional fermented soya product in Japan. Itihiki-natto is an aged product of the *Bacillus* fermentation of the steamed soybean. Sufu is a Chinese product prepared from fermented soybean.

Table 6: Country wise usage of different probiotic products

Fermented products	Substrates used	Sensory property	Type of products	Microorganisms used	Country
Ambali	Millet, rice	Acidic,	Pancake	LAB	India
Batura	Wheat flour	Bread	Pancake	LAB, yeasts	India
Ben-saalga	Pearl millet	Gruel Weaning	Food	LAB, yeasts	Ghana
Chilra	Wheat, barley, buck wheat	Dough	Staple	LAB, yeasts	India
Idli	Rice and black gram	Mildly acidic, soft, spongy	Breakfast food	LAB, yeasts	India, Srilanka, Malaysia
Jalebi	Wheat flour	Crispy, sweet	Deep fried snacks	LAB, yeasts	India, Pakistan, Nepal
Kinky	Maize	Acidic, solid	Steamed, staple	LAB, yeasts	Ghana
Maheu	Maize, sorghum, millet	Sour, nonalcoholic	Beverage	LAB	South Africa
Mawe	Maize	Sour, nonalcoholic	Porridge Yeasts,	LAB	Togo, Benin
Naan	Wheat flour	Baked bread	Staple	LAB, yeasts	
Natto	Soybean	Alkaline	Breakfast	Bacillus natto	India, Afghanistan Pakistan
Ogi	Maize, sorghum, millet	Acidic	Staple porridge	LAB, yeasts	Nigeria
Pizza dough	Wheat	Leavened dough	Used as base	Baker's yeast	worldwide
Puda/pudla	Maize, Bengal gram	Pancake	Snack food	LAB, yeasts	India
Rabadi	Cereals, pulses with cow milk	Thick product with Milk	Drink slight Acidic	LAB, Yeasts	India, Pakistan
Sourdough	Wheat, Rye Leavened	bread	Breakfast	LAB, yeasts	Australia, Europe
Trahana	Rice, wheat, soybean and milk	Sweet and sour soup	Yeasts,	LAB	Turkey
Uji	Maize, sorghum, millet	Sour	Staple	LAB	Kenya, Tanzania

Source: Champagne (2009)

Table 7: Probiotic products with targeted health benefits available in the USA

Infant diarrhea	*L. rhamnosus* GG Culturelle (capsule) (aka —Immunitas™")	Danimals (drinkable yogurt) Dan Active (fermented milk)
L. casei DN-114001		
Inflammatory bowel conditions IBD	*Lactobacillus* strains *Bifidobacterium* strains, 4 *Lactobacillus* strains and *S. thermophilus*	8-strain; combination of 3
VSL#3 (powder)	Antibiotic associated diarrhea; *C. difficile*	
S. boulardii, Florastor (powder)	*L. rhamnosus* GG Culturelle (capsule)	Danimals (drinkable yogurt)
L. casei DN114001 Dan Active (fermented milk) Activia (yogurt)	Gut transit time B. animalis DN-173 010 (aka Keeping healthy *L. reuteri* ATCC 55730 Stony field yogurt	Bifidus regularis™" *L. casei* DN-114001 Dan Active (fermented milk)
L. casei Shirota Yakult *L. rhamnosus* GG Culturelle (capsule) Thermophilus (most strains)	Allergy (atopic dermatitis) Danimals (drikable yogurt) All yogurts with live, active cultures Reuteri drops	(in infants) Lactose intolerance *L. bulgaricus* and/or *S. Colic* in infants *L. reuteri* ATCC 55730
Immune support *B. lactis* HN019 aka Smoothie Strain sold as an *B. lactis* Bb-12 Good Start Natural Cultures (infant supplement products - contact Chr.	HOWARU™ or DR10 Ingredient for dairy and supplement formula) Nestle Strain also Hansens (800-558-0802)	Naked Juice Probiotic Juice Products - contact Danisco An ingredient for dairy and sold as *L. casei* DN114001 Dan Active (fermented milk)
L. rhamnosus GG Culturelle (capsule) Vaginal applications *L. rhamnosus* GR-1, *L. reuteri* Irritable bowel syndrome symptoms	Danimals (drikable yogurt) RC-14 *B. infantis* 35264 (aka)	*L. reuteri* ATCC 55730 Stonyfield yogurt Fem-Dophilus (capsules)

Source: CRDF. California Dairy Research Foundation (2015).

The fermented dairy products are generally considered to be safe and nutritious. The beneficial effect of fermented milk products may be further enhanced by supplementation of probiotic bacteria which should have a good shelf life.

The probiotic products available in the market today are dairy products (Boasso *et al.*, 2007). Milk contains a rich source of nutrients and thus serves as a good media for the growth of probiotic strains. The base for the production of dairy products is milk, which has a typical composition of H" 87.4%, H" 4.7% lactose, H" 3.8% fat, H" 3.3% protein, H" 0.2% citrate, and H" 0.6% minerals. The pH of the milk is usually between 6.5 and 6.7. The protein fraction is composed of 80% casein and 20% whey proteins (Schlimme *et al.*, 1995). Fermented milk is one of the dairy products obtained by the use of appropriate probiotic bacteria which results in lowering of pH with or without coagulation of fermented milk (Abdelbasset and Djamila, 2008). All dairy products need to have a good shelf life.

Usually the LAB cultures used as starter cultures for the preparation of dairy products include *Lactobacillus, Bifidobacteria, Pediococcus* and *Lactococcus etc*. The probiotic food supplements that contain these LAB strains are one of the important classes of functional foods. Champagne (2009) has looked into the technological challenges when probiotic bacteria are added to food matrix.

7
ANIMAL AND CLINICAL STUDIES

Antibiotic Resistance and Gene transfer

It is important that probiotic strains should be assessed for their phenotypical antibiotic resistance and potential to transfer resistance gene as otherwise they cannot be used in food (BgVV, 2000; Vankerckhoven et al., 2008). It is vital to do research on characterization of acquired resistance mechanisms and transferability of resistance genes and on methods for determining transferability.

Most of the infant formulas are known to have probiotic strains which possess acquired antibiotic resistance gene. *Lb.reuteri* ATCC 55730 has two antibiotic resistance genes: tetracycline and lincosamide (Kastner et al., 2006).

Elimination of antibiotic resistance by selective removal or curing of plasmids can be an approach to solve this problem.

Deleterious Metabolic Activities: D-Lactic acid

D-Lactic acid is produced by some *Lactobacilli* which are utilized in infant formulae. L (+) lactic acid is naturally there in the human body and gets degraded. D-lactic acid is degraded via the enzyme D-2- hydroxyl acid dehydrogenase (Uribarri et al., 1998). D-lactic acid is taken up from the colon and is then secreted out with urine. In a safety study of FAO/ WHO in infants it was concluded that neither D-lactic acid nor DL-lactic acid should be used in infant foods (FAO/WHO, 1973). It was found that there was no elevation of D-lactic acid in the blood of infants which were given *L.reuteri* ATCC55730 at a dose of 10^8 cfu/d for 12 months.

Addition of probiotics in infant food has shown benefits in the treatment of allergy, NEC and acute diarrhea. However, it was seen that the results are strain specific and are dependent on the dose given. The probiotic to be given should be checked for its efficacy and safety in the final product composition before bringing it to the market. The dosage according to FAO/WHO is live microorganisms which when administered in adequate amounts confer a health benefit on the host (Agostoni *et al.*, 2004). Critical identification of the strains to be used in commercial products is highly desirable (Huys *et al.*, 2006).

The diseases are influenced by nutrition later in life. Probiotics offer beneficial effects on the host. The great variability of the intestinal microbiota might indicate that different bacteria play different roles in the symbiosis between microbiota and the host. Studies by modern techniques may identify and quantify the intestinal bacteria and the complex ecosystem. Modulation of the immune system and intestinal resistance offers an opportunity for prevention of infectious and immune related diseases.

To prevent allergies during the entire life it may be important to modulate the developing immune system. There have been many clinical studies where consumption of probiotics have shown health improvement like eczema (Kalliomaki *et al.*, 2001; Marteau *et al.*, 2002) and reduction in antibiotic associated diarrhoea (Plummer *et al.*, 2004).

A study suggested that the anecdotal benefits of probiotic therapies are beneficial for preventing secondary infections which is a common complication of antibiotic therapy. Keeping the immune system primed by eating foods with —good bacteria (probiotic) may help to counteract the negative effects of sickness and antibiotics. It is possible that antibiotics turn the immune system —off "where as the probiotics bring it back on —idle", and more able to quickly react to new infections.

Clinical trials have demonstrated that probiotics may decrease the incidence of respiratory tract infections (Hatakka *et al.*, 2001) and dental caries in children (Näse *et al.*, 2001). LAB foods and supplements have been shown positive in the treatment and prevention of acute diarrhea, and in decreasing the severity and duration of rotavirus infection in children and travelers' diarrhea in adults (Reid *et al.*, 2003)

LAB supplements have been found to modulate inflammatory and hypersensitivity responses, an observation thought to be at least in part due to the regulation of cytokine function (Reid *et al.*, 2003). Clinical studies suggest that probiotics can prevent reoccurrences of inflammatory bowel disease in adults, as well as improve milk allergies (Kirjavainen *et al.*, 2003). Several *in vivo* studies have demonstrated that some *Lactobacillus* strains can improve the antioxidant status of rats and humans (Kaizu *et al.*, 1993; Kullisaar *et al.*, 2003). Therefore, many investigations have focused on antioxidant properties of lactic acid bacteria and their role in health and disease recently (Ito *et al.*, 2003; Kim *et al.*, 2006). Crooks *et al.* (2012) have written a clinical review on the importance of probiotics in critical care.

There are only few studies about the effects of *Lactobacillus* on the antioxidant status of pigs (Wang *et al.*, 2009), especially on weaning piglets.

The *in vivo* trial was carried out to estimate the effects of *Lactobacillus plantarum* ZLP001 supplementation in weaning piglets. It was demonstrated that weaning in piglets is related to oxidative stress (Sauerwein *et al.*, 2007). This stress can result in reduced performance and increased susceptibility to disease and death (Hampson, 1994; Cromwell, 2002).

Ito *et al.* (2001) have studied the antioxidative effects of live Bifidobacteria on lipid peroxidation in the colonic mucosa of rats. It was found that the level of lipid peroxide decreased. Oral administration of *B.bifidum* strain for two weeks significantly decreased the level of lipid peroxidation in the colonic mucosa of iron overloaded mice. Kullisar *et al.* (2003) have studied the effect of fermented goat's milk with *Lactobacillus fermentum* ME-3 on antiatherogenicity in healthy subjects and prolonged resistance of lipoprotein fraction to oxidation and lowered the level of peroxidized lipoproteins. The fecal concentrations of *L. casei* DN 114 001Rif reported by Yuki *et al.* (1999) are substantially higher than the concentration of *L. casei* strain Shirota, estimated at 7 log cfu/g⁻1 of feces with a similar inoculum, suggesting lower survival abilities of the latter strain. The fecal population of *L.casei* DN-114 001Rif, corresponding to about 0.1% of the autochthonous microbiota, may be a key factor in its probiotic activities (Berg, 1996 and Marteau *et al.*, 1993). The transit marker persisted longer, reaching a plateau from 2 to 6 h after ingestion. The highest concentration of *L. casei* DN 114 001Rif detected in this compartment represented 10 to 100 times more bacteria than the resident microbiota (Berg, 1996), and it largely exceeded the concentration of probiotics that was previously suggested by some authors for the recovery of a clinical effect (6 log cfu /ml^{-1} in the small bowel (Marteau *et al.*, 1993). Cazaubiel and Cazaubiel (2010) have studied the psychotropic properties of a probiotic formulation on rat and human subjects.

8
ROLE OF PACKAGING TO ENHANCE SHELF LIFE OF PROBIOTIC PRODUCTS

Probiotics are measured in colony forming units (cfu). CFUs are generally measured in the millions or billions per serving. Probiotics are most commonly beneficial bacteria, but can also be friendly fungal or other organisms, that are typically freeze dried to stabilize them in an inert state during storage and production. Then their continued stability and viability, as measured by CFU counts when cultured, is dependent on limiting their exposure to stimulating environmental conditions such as temperature and moisture. Besides refrigeration, this protection can be done by packaging in glass or by adding freshness packets that helps to absorb and reduce moisture in the package.

Temperature plays a role in the stability of probiotics. Colder air holds less moisture and is not in the ideal temperature range for the bacteria to commonly grow and thrive, thus inhibiting reactivation of the dormant organisms by depriving them of the warmth and moisture that represent their ideal growing conditions. High heat can also degrade the viability of these organisms.

Even under ideal storage conditions, the number of colony forming units will slowly decline with time. For example, packing in glass gives a drop of 5% per month in the cell number of the probiotic under non-refrigerated conditions. Refrigeration has been seen to prolong the potency and viability of most probiotics to maintain higher counts over a longer period of time.

In order to meet label claims for probiotic CFU numbers, manufacturers generally add an overage to allow for the natural decline in numbers over time. We test to assure that the product meets specifications and label claims in terms of potency (CFUs) at the time of manufacture. Stability studies utilizing the strains, potencies and designated packaging for a specific product are also done as needed to generate data to calculate an experimental stability curve that predicts changing CFU counts throughout the shelf life of the product. However, the actual rate of change depends on the environment to which the product is exposed especially if not kept in refrigerated conditions.

The rate of decline in viable CFU numbers can increase if a probiotic product is held in conditions that are very warm or moist, especially after opening when moisture can more easily get into the package. Because of the extreme variability of the seasonal weather and environmental conditions that a product may experience, and duration of these exposures, it's not possible to precisely predict potency and shelf life accurately for every person's situation across a wide geographical area. In some cases, it could happen that adverse conditions may lower probiotic counts below label claim.

According to the proposed concept on the efficacy of probiotic application, the probiotic bacteria must be viable at the time of consumption to achieve beneficial function. Official standards for the minimum suggested level for probiotics in the food to attain this viability require a minimum of 10^6-10^7 cfu/g, which have been introduced by several food organizations worldwide (Talwalkar and Kailasapathy, 2004). Drying is widely used as a means of preservation of bacterial cells. Because high water activity dramatically decreases the viability of probiotics, removal of water can effectively extend the shelf life of probiotic products. Drying is widely used as a means of preservation of bacterial cells. Because high water activity dramatically decreases the viability of probiotics, removal of water can effectively extend the shelf life of probiotic products. Freeze-drying is another practicable method to improve the viability of probiotics is to immobilize the bacteria in an external protective matrix, which can improve their resistance to adverse conditions and facilitate better survival in specific food products (Adhikari, *et al.*, 2003; Godward and Kailasapathy, 2003). Freeze-drying is a common method used to incorporate probiotics in foods. However, the viability of freeze-dried probiotic bacteria is affected during processing and storage. Freeze-dried probiotic organisms are protected by adding cryoprotectants, and the identification of protective agents that enhance cellular survival during storage and application in food is the key challenge (Hubalek, 2003). The technique of micro-encapsulation based on complex (w/o/w) dispersion offers several advantages for the immobilization of probiotics. Zhoa and Zhang (2005) studied for *L.brevis* when supplemented with sucrose, trehalose and sorbitol. In skim milk, sucrose and trehalose are most commonly used industrially. Scientists have (Lislie *et al.*, 1995; Hubalek, 2003; Carvalho *et al.*, 2003b) reported that lactose had high colony count during freeze drying which was higher than that of sucrose, sorbitol and trehalose. Chavarri *et al.* (1988) found that lactose (2.0×10^8 cfu/ml) provide higher viability of *L. lactis* during storage at 20°C to -70°C when glycerol was utilized. Bruno and Shah (2003) have studied the viability of *Bifidobacteria* after freeze drying and showed that the culture survival rate was 46.2 to 75.1%. Champagne *et al.* (1996) reported that gelatin, xanthin gum and maltodextrin were used as a protective media on *Lactobacillus casei, Bifidobacterium longum, Lactococcus lactis* and *Streptococcus thermophilus* during freeze drying. To dry at low temperature, viability of starter cultures can be improved by adding sugar sorbitol as a protective agent. The vacuum dried cells have very high storage stability under protective agents. A significant change in viability after drying was not found in cells storage at low humidity and temperatures (aw of 0.1, 0.2 and 0.3; 4°C) for a year (Santivarangkna *et al.*, 2007). Carvalho *et al.* (2003a) have studied the effect of different sugars when added to the growth and drying medium upon thermotolerance and survival during storage of freeze-dried *Lactobacillus delbrueckii* spp., *bulgaricus.* Shobharani and Agrawal (2010) have shown the enhancement of cell stability and viability of probiotic *Leuconostoc mesenteroides* MTCC 5209 on freeze drying to be used in food formulation. Champagne *et al.* (1991) have written a good review on the freeze drying of lactic acid bacteria. Sudha *et al.* (2006) studied the stability and viability of a local probiotic isolate *Pediococcus pentosaceous* (MTCC 5151) under induced gastrointestinal tract conditions by checking the colony forming units. Chandramouli *et al.* (2004) found significant increase in the viable number of culture *L.acidophilus* when encapsulated in alginate at pH 2.0. *Lactobacilli* immobilized in alginate beads survived at higher rate when incubated in simulated gastric fluid (Lian *et al.*, 2003). Krasaekoopt *et al.* (2004) found microencapsulated cells of *L. acidophilus* in alginate beads survived well even after the incubation period in simulated gastric juice. Several reports are available for the tolerance of lactic acid bacteria to high bile salt environment (Conway *et al.*, 1987; Lee and Heo, 2000; Sultana *et al.*, 2000). Guerin *et al.* (2003) reported that the *Bifidobacteria* immobilized in polysaccharide protein gel beads were able to withstand exposure of 2 and 4% bile salt concentrations. Lian *et al.* (2003) studied the viability of microencapsulated *Bifidobacteria* in simulated gastric juice and bile solution. Viable lactic acid bacteria of probiotic foods have several scientifically established and/or clinically proved health effects, such as reduction and prevention of diarrhea's of different origin, improvement of the intestinal microbial balance by antimicrobial activity, alleviation of lactose intolerance symptoms, prevention of food allergy, enhancement of immune potency, and antitumorigenic activities (McFarland, 2000; Andersson *et al.*, 2001; Salminen, 2001). Giulio *et al.* (2005) have studied the improvement of viability in lactic acid bacteria by using cryoprotectants. Miao *et al.* (2008) studied the effect of disaccharides on survival of probiotics during freeze drying. Moreover, some studies have shown that some of the lactic acid bacteria possess antioxidative activity (Kaizu *et al.*, 1993; Peuhkuri *et al.*, 1996; and

Kullisaar *et al.*, 2002). They are able to decrease the risk of accumulation of reactive oxygen species in a host organism and could potentially be used in probiotic food supplements to reduce oxidative stress. In a previous study (Kullisaar *et al.*, 2002) it was reported that *Lactobacillus fermentum* strain ME-3 (DSM 14241) has high antimicrobial and antioxidative activity. In healthy volunteers, it has been demonstrated that the consumption of fermented milk containing this *Lactobacillus fermentum* strain exhibited antioxidative and antiatherogenic effects (Kullisaar *et al.*, 2003). Dinesh Kumar and Agrawal (2008) have shown the therapeutic importance of probiotic fermented milk using a native isolate of *Pediococcus pentosaceous* MTCC 5151.

Probiotic foods have gained interest in recent years due to the various health benefits it provides to the human health. To get the maximum benefits, several functional properties of the food should be maintained throughout its shelf storage. In designing probiotic foods, many constraints like viability of cells, tolerance of the bacteria to the gut environment have to be known. With the development of science and technology, alternative materials like plastics have emerged either to replace natural and traditional materials with a benefit of cost reduction purpose, to cater to certain applications which were not available with those of traditional materials.

In the modern times product marketers knows precisely the time period (shelf life) over which the package is required to preserve the product. The marketers, now, with the use of plastics is in a position to select the right structure and get the desired protection and preservation capabilities required for the product and the market. Stronger packages such as metal containers and glass bottles were used for quite some time for preserving the product as long as possible. With the development of technology, modern packaging materials have been available to protect and preserve the food products.

To evaluate the shelf life of probiotic fermented milk in different packaging materials studies have been undertaken by various scientists. The study comprised of inoculum size of probiotic lactic acid bacteria in milk samples packed in different packaging materials which were allowed for fermentation. The samples were analyzed for different functional properties during the shelf storage of three days. This includes analysis of pH, volatile compounds formed which have therapeutic importance, antimicrobial activity against toxic food pathogen and antibiotic susceptibility.

It is important to check the shelf life of the probiotic fermented milk in different packaging materials and establish the best packaging material that can be used for the shelf storage of probiotic fermented milk along with maximum antimicrobial activity against toxic food pathogens (Mezaini *et al.*, 2009). India is also becoming an attractive destination for investments in this sector. The growing health-consciousness in newer generation has paved the way for varieties of weight reducing, low-cholesterol, high fibre and nutrient-rich food products.

Good Packaging is needed to perform four basic functions as follows:

- Protection
- Communication
- Convenience
- Containment

In olden days traditionally metal containers, bamboo baskets, wooden containers and jute sacks were used for packaging. Later steel container was used. With the development of science and technology, the alternative materials like plastics have emerged to replace the traditional packaging.

Even, in plastics, there are a variety of materials, which are used for packaging applications. The important food grade plastics, which find large packaging applications, are HDPE, PP, LDPE, PVC, Polyester, Polystyrene *etc*. These are used for building the body structure of the packagers, while other polymers are often used, in less thickness, as coating to improve the functional properties of basic packaging.

Thus, the advantage of plastics is in the range of mechanical barrier and other properties it offers and also the feasibility of tailoring a structure required to meet processing the product protection, preservation and distribution needs. Consumers increasingly demand food, which retains the natural flavor, color, texture and contains fewer additives such as preservatives.

In response to these needs, one of the most important recent developments in the food industry has been the development of minimal processing technologies or smart packaging.

This is designed to limit the impact of processing on nutritional and sensory quality and to preserve food without the use of synthetic additives. Smart packaging offers the additional functionalities depending upon the type of product.

These include:

- To retain the integrity of a product
- Prevent food spoilage
- Enhance product attributes such as look, taste, aroma, *etc*.

- Respond actively to changes in the product and package environment
- Communicate product information, product history or condition to the user
- Indicate seal integrity or confirm product authenticity *etc.*

As mentioned in Encyclopedia Britannica: — "smart packaging offer properties to maintain the special needs of certain foods".

For eg: packages made with oxygen absorbing materials remove oxygen from the inside of the package and protects oxygen-sensitive products from oxidation.

Therefore, intelligent packaging could be defined as a packaging system that is capable of carrying out intelligent functions (such as sensing, detecting, tracing, recording and communicating) to facilitate decision making to extend shelf life, improve quality, enhance safety, provide information, and warn about possible problems (www.pdq.wur.nl).

Intelligent packaging systems have components that sense the environment and process the information and allow the action to protect the product by conducting the communication functions. Hence it has a good potential for use in food and beverage products due to an increase in the demand for diagnostic packaging in response to the consumer desire for more information about freshness of foods, and need for track and trace systems.

Viability during Processing and Storage

In Brazil, it is required that the fermented milks must have a viability of LAB and *Bifidobacterium* to at least 10^7 and 10^6 CFU/g or mL, respectively at the end of the product shelf life (MAPA, 2007). Optimum growth of probiotics is seen at temperatures within 40-42°C in the fermented foods. When the temperatures are above 45-50°C during processing then it is known to be detrimental to probiotic survival (Tripathi and Giri, 2014). The viability during storage, processing and survival when in intestinal transit are the main criteria for the selection of any strain of probiotic bacteria (Talwalkar and Kailasapathy, 2004). When the probiotic culture is added to any product the physiological state of the probiotic cultures also plays a major factor affecting the overall culture viability. In this respect, the induction of stress responses on the probiotic strains can attribute a dramatic effect on the ability of the cultures to survive processing (such as freeze drying and spray drying) and gastric transit (Ross *et al.*, 2005).

Acid stress significantly affects the viability of a culture (Shah, 2007). Consequently, dairy products are preferred for use as carriers of probiotic strains for enhancement of microbial survival in gastric juice, due to buffering or protective effect (Ross *et al.*, 2005). It has been observed that *Bifidobacterium* cultures are less acid tolerant than *Lactobacillus* cultures and have less tolerance to human gastric juice. Tolerance to an acidic environment is important in fermented foods (Ross *et al.*, 2005; Mättö *et al.*, 2006). Rao *et al.* (2007) studied the role of oxygen scavengers in improving the stability and viability of *Pediococcus pentosaceous*.

Viability of probiotic microorganisms in food products is mainly influenced during production, processing and storage which include food parameters (molecular oxygen, water activity, presence of salt, sugar and chemicals like hydrogen peroxide, bacteriocins, artificial flavouring and colouring agents), processing parameters (heat treatment, incubation temperature, cooling rate of the product, packaging materials, storage methods, scale of production) and microbiological parameters (strains of probiotics, rate and proportion of inoculation) (Tripathi and Giri, 2014). Oxygen content and redox potential (microaerophilic and anaerobic) also play a vital role (Shah, 2007). In aerobic conditions lactic acid bacteria generate more hydrogen peroxide due to the action of flavoprotein-containing oxidases, Nicotinamide Adenine Dinucleotide oxidases (NADH) and Superoxide Dismutase (SOD) than they do under anaerobic conditions (Miller and Britigan, 1997; Kulisaar *et al.*, 2002). The oxygen content affects the probiotics in the following ways (i) toxicity to some cells, (ii) toxic peroxides are formed (iii) oxidation of components produce free radicals like fats (Korbekandi *et al.*, 2011; Tripathi and Giri, 2014). One solution is the addition of ascorbic acid (vitamin C), which can act as an oxygen scavenger (Shah, 2000). Refrigeration is ideal for storing probiotics. But if that is not possible, it is best to keep the package in a cool, dry place to maintain good stability. Unfortunately, many people tend to keep their supplements in the kitchen or bathroom, which are notorious for being warm, moist and known to shorten the shelf life of many kinds of supplements. Those conditions are ideal for bacterial and mold growth which means that the probiotics will first tend to activate but then die off more quickly than expected since they are not yet in the human body where they have a chance to live, grow, and thrive. In these adverse conditions, probiotics may lose potency more rapidly than anticipated and thus may not meet label claims for CFU counts that are calculated based on a cool, dry place. On the other hand, refrigerating probiotic products will enhance viability and shelf life. Kailaspathy and Chin (2000) have studied the survival and therapeutic potential of probiotic organisms with reference to *Lactobacillus acidophilus* and *Bifidobacterium* spp.

In testing designed to mimic exposures during transportation in a hot climate, a sealed probiotic formula exposed to a temperature of over 122° F for 24 hours still met label claim for CFU content. This indicates that this level of heat over that time period was not enough to kill many of the organisms in the package, so it would take even harsher conditions to rapidly degrade the potency of the specific probiotic product.

There is some evidence that even non-viable probiotic organisms left in the package after being exposed to unfavorable conditions may have some utility in gut health. For example, it is hypothesized that they may take up ecological space on the intestinal walls, which may help to prevent the growth of opportunistic organisms vying for that same space. For example, inactivated *Lactobacillus plantarum* has been shown in clinical studies to support our natural immunity to foreign substances (so-called acquired immunity).

The stability of a probiotic formula tested at the time of manufacture depends on a combination of factors. Variations in packaging, temperature, and humidity affect the viability of probiotic products before they are consumed. Protective factors that help to preserve the freshness and viability of the probiotic strains in a supplement include refrigeration, resistant packaging, and storage in a cool, dry place.

Freezing is an important factor which affects the viability of probiotic culture. The freezing step in food processing is especially critical as it negatively affects both viability and physiological state of the bacteria. The properties of the cellular membrane are affected due to low temperature. During freezing, the liquid phase moves to a liquid-crystalline phase and therefore membrane fluidity is reduced causing cellular death. Crystallization of water causes the solutes to concentrate, which induces some osmotic damage (McGann, 1978; Foschino *et al.*, 1995; Beal *et al.*, 2001). Survival in freezing conditions and storage varies with the strain (Fonseca *et al.*, 2000). It was observed that small spherical cells of *Enterococci* were more stable during freezing and freeze-drying than the large rods of *Lactobacilli* (Fonseca *et al.*, 2000). It has been reported by Senz *et al.* (2015) that among the *Lactobacilli* higher stability is observed in short rods than elongated rods on freeze-drying. Supplementation of adjuvants to probiotic cultures can improve their viability during manufacture. Glucose was found good to energize cells upon exposure to acid (Corcoran *et al.*, 2005) and cryoprotectants such as glycerol or inulin for improving survivability during freeze-drying (Fonseca *et al.*, 2000; Carvalho *et al.*, 2004).

Bacterio (phages) usually spoil the fermented foods particularly dairy fermentations, resulting in slow vats, low quality, inconsistent products and even complete fermentation failure (Mahony and Sinderen, 2015). Phage-host interactions can be obtained byphages infecting LAB (Mahony and Sinderen, 2015). A number of strategies for strain diversity, bacteriophage-insensitive mutants and plasmids bearing phage-resistance mechanisms (Barrangou *et al.*, 2007) have been designed recently and have been implemented to reduce both the presence of phages in the dairy industry and their economic impact on fermentation processes (Briggiler *et al.*, 2014).

Bacteria have developed many natural defense mechanisms that target diverse steps of the phage life cycle, that blocks adsorption, prevents DNA injection, restricts the incoming DNA and abortive infection systems (Barrangou *et al.*, 2007). Two methodologies were used to isolate phage-resistant mutants namely the Agar Plate (AP) and the Secondary Culture (SC) methods (Briggiler *et al.* 2011).

Clustered Regularly Interspaced Short Palindromic Repeats (CRISPR) is the loci which are hyper variabally distributed in bacteria. This provides acquired immunity against foreign genetic elements. CRISPRs are DNA repeats consisting of short and highly conserved repeats, interspaced by variable sequences called spacers, and are often times adjacent to cas (CRISPR-associated) genes (Sorek *et al.*, 2008). The CRISPR-cas system may accordingly be exploited as a virus defense mechanism and also potentially used to reduce the dissemination of mobile genetic elements and the acquisition of undesirable traits such as antibiotic resistance genes and virulence markers. From a phage evolution perspective, the integrated phage sequences within CRISPR loci may also provide additional anchor points to facilitate recombination during subsequent phage infections, thereby increasing the gene pool to which phages have access (Barrangou *et al.*, 2007). A key distinguishing feature in LAB is the CRISPR loci for phylogenetic and genome evolution. It also provides immunity against foreign genetic elements which are involved in the microbes propensity to survive phage predation and to adapt that environment. Surya Chandra Rao *et al.* (2007) have studied the role of oxygen scavengers in improving the stability and viability of probiotic lactic acid bacteria. Shobharani and Agrawal (2010) studied the interception of quorum sensing signal molecule by furanone to enhance the shelf life of fermented milk.

Contribution to Sensory Properties in Probiotic foods

LAB usually degrades proteins (Lopez-Kleine *et al.*, 2011). There is a Change in acid production and proteolysis in strains from naturalsources (Franciosi *et al.*, 2009).

Sulphur compounds are usually formed during proteolysis. Due to the accumulation of hydrophobic peptides (i.e. peptides rich in proline) bitterness, is caused which affects the quality of Gouda and Cheddar cheeses (Smit *et al.*, 2005; Savijoki *et al.*, 2006). Ong and Shah (2008) have worked on the influence of probiotic *Lactobacillus acidophilus* and *L. helveticus* on proteolysis, organic acid profiles, and ACE-inhibitory activity of cheddar cheeses which were ripened at 4, 8, and 12 degrees. It has been seen that starter culture and the flavour in fermented sausages are correlated (Sidira *et al.*, 2015). Flavours are most of the times formed by biotransformation which are either produced by lipid hydrolysis or autoxidation and also by proteolysis and transformation of amino acids to aromatic compounds and carbohydrate metabolism (Ammor *et al.*, 2007). Probiotics with proteolytic activity increased the generation of peptides with antioxidant potential and antimutagenic properties (Sah *et al.*, 2014). Occurrence of exopolysaccharides (EPS) is well documented in all organisms (viz. animals, plants, fungi and bacteria). These are involved in various biological functions for the storage of energy (starch), cell wall architecture (cellulose) or in cellular communication (Raposo *et al.*, 2013). These are categorized under GRAS status (Ahmed*et al.*, 2013; Yang *et al.*, 2014) and therefore can be utilized as a food additive for improving the texture of food products with improved appearance, stability and rheological properties (De Vuyst *et al.*, 2001). It also improves functions of defense mechanism against bacteriophages by preventing their adsorption (Lamothe and Boullier, 2002). According to Kodali *et al.* (2009) *Lactobacillus* produces EPS molecules in relatively large amounts (>100 mg/l) media enriched with glucose. The viscosity and biological activity of an EPS depends on its molecular weight, sugar composition and primary structure. Liu *et al.* (2010) and Nikolic *et al.* (2012) observed that EPS secreted by *B. licheniformis* and *L. paraplantarum* have immunomodulatory capacity, immunosuppressive and anti-inflammatory actions. Antitumor effects, hypocholesterolemic activity and enhanced colonization of probiotic bacteria in the gastrointestinal tract have also been observed (Welman and Maddox, 2003). LABS have evolved mechanisms to support various concentrations of NaCl that generally involve the absorption or synthesis of a limited number of solutes (Bremer and Kramer, 2000). Osmotic stress may become the major inhibiting factor for bacterial growth and fermentation (Ge *et al.*, 2001). Reale *et al.* (2015) added information on intra species variability in osmotolerance of *L. casei, L. paracasei* and *L. rhamnosus* which is an important criterion for the selection of strains for technological applications. In particular, several strains isolated from cheese and human feces appeared to be very tolerant of high NaCl concentrations and are worth investigating for their performance in fermented foods. Ammor *et al.* (2007) also affirmed good ability of a starter culture to compete with the natural microbiota of a raw material (sausage) and for expected metabolic activities by its growth rate and survival in the conditions prevailing in the sausage, including high salt concentrations ranging from 2% to 15% in the final product. Majchrzak *et al.* (2010) have found that the conventional and probiotic yoghurts differ sensorily but not in consumer acceptance.

In some products such as kefir and some cheeses like Goudagas are produced (Leite *et al.*, 2013; Pedersen *et al.*, 2013) by lactic acid bacteria. Gas production is known to increase the number and/or size of holes in semi-hard cheeses. Eye formation in cheese depends on gas formation, gas diffusion, the presence of eye-forming nuclei, pH and elasticity of the cheese body, as well as technological parameters (Fröhlich-Wyder *et al.*, 2002). Anaerobic production of CO_2 by *Lactobacilli* has been found in cheese (Tammam *et al.*, 2000). Heterofermentative LAB in sausage production are not good as large amounts of carbon dioxide is formed that forms holes of different sizes in the product also production of acetic acid causes pungent off-flavors (Buckenhüskes, 1993; Ammor *et al.*, 2007).

Aroma, flavor and taste make any food item very important and attractive to consume. Aroma compounds play a major role for perceiving flavor. This is important for consumers (Chen *et al.*, 2013). Diacetyl (2,3-butanedione) is a volatile product of citrate metabolism produced by lactic acid bacteria, and when taken in conjunction with the lactic acid and textural effects, it enhances the sensorial profile of fermented foods (Rincon-Delgadillo *et al.*, 2012; Xião and Lu, 2014). It can also inhibit pathogenic micro-organisms by penetrating the targeted bacterial membranes and interfering with essential metabolic functions. High diacetyl levels are associated with a flavor imbalance, bitter taste and harsh aroma (Clarke *et al.*, 2009), but it is used as an ingredient in the formulation of many food products such as cottage cheese, margarine, vegetable oil spreads, processed cheese and sour cream to increase the levels of the naturally occurring buttery aroma associated with fermentation (Rincon-Delgadillo *et al.*, 2012). Renu Agrawal *et al.* (2000) have studied the flavour profile of idli batter prepared from defined microbial starter cultures over a shelf life. They have also discussed how with time duration toxic volatiles are formed which make the product unacceptable.

9
MARKET TREND ON PROBIOTIC AROUND THE WORLD

What new research is needed, what trials and how will the ultimate consumer and Industry benefit?

In Brazil, the sales of functional foods amounts to US $ 500 million per year representing about 1% of the total sale of the Brazilian food processing industry. According to a report the interests are mainly for dairy products, nutraceuticals and soy-based products. ABIA forecasts a substantial growth of 4.5-5% for this segment of the market (Stanton *et al.*, 2001). In order to exert the health benefits beyond inherent basic nutrition, it is necessary that the activity of the probiotic culture should be maintained at very high levels during the shelf life of the product. There is a lot of interest with the microbiologists and food scientists around the globe who are involved with academics, industrially employed dieticians and nutritionists. Regulators in U.S. Food and Drug Administration, U.S. Department of Agriculture and people in state and city health departments are also looking ahead for probiotic foods as there is a lot of interest in the real and/or postulated health benefits and inhibition in disease treatment. It is observed that a probiotic culture should have oxygen tolerance, acid and bile tolerance and heat tolerance for human consumption. Many scientists are working in this direction to get good probiotic cultures. Commonly used cultures are *Lactobacillus* sp. and *Bifidobacterium* sp. (Stanton *et al.*, 2003 a, b).

The factors responsible for the inclination of consumers towards functional foods are baby health conscious movement, chronic health diseases in aged people, changes in food regulations, market opportunity, increased health care costs, changing consumer demands and social attitudes. New opportunities will add value to the existing products with higher profits (Anonymous 2002, 2006, 2010). Presently, the main emphasis is on clinical applications (benefits and/or lack thereof) as well as future biomedical therapeutic uses in animal model studies focused on therapies and data for the probiotics to be used as complementary and alternative medicines. Product development with probiotics is on the forefront. Information on pre-and probiotics as important sources of micro-and macronutrients aid in the development of methods of bio-modification of dietary plant molecules for health promotion. Pre-and probiotics provide defense system for the selection of food for individual consumption based on health needs and current status (Anonymous, 2011). It is assumed that global probiotic market will exceed US$29.8 billion by 2016. The market is set to witness impressive growth as consumers become more conscious about their health and switch to preventive healthcare due to rising healthcare cost. Sharma *et al.* (2014) have discussed antibiotic resistance among the commercially available probiotic.

10

FUTURE IMPLICATIONS OF PROBIOTICS

In spite of the problems with dosage and viability of probiotic strains, a lot more work is required for industry standardization and safety issues. However, it is noted that probiotics have considerable potential against many pathogenic and other diseases. A wide range of clinical trials are still needed to standardize and optimize the conditions. Ongoing basic research will continue to identify and characterize existing strains of probiotics, identifying strain-specific outcomes, determine optimal doses needed for certain results and assess their stability through processing and digestion. Gene technology will certainly play a role in developing new strains, with gene sequencing allowing for an increased understanding of mechanisms and functionality of probiotics. In addition to such basic research, industry centered research will focus on prolonging the shelf-life and likelihood of survival through the intestinal tract, optimizing adhesion capacity and developing proper production, handling and packaging procedures to ensure that the desired benefits are delivered to the consumer. In time to come, new probiotic food products will enter the market which may include energy bars, cereals, juices, infant formulas, different kind of cheeses as well as disease-specific medical foods. The establishment of standards to identity probiotic in food products will serve to accelerate the development and availability of these food products (Parvez et al., 2006b).

Probiotics for Specific Target Groups

Current probiotics have been selected based on the probiotic properties stated earlier in this book. To refine the selection criteria, understanding of the mechanisms of probiotic action is necessary. A lot of work is underway on the mechanistic of probiotics. This will make it possible to select future strains with more specific characteristics, to suit the needs of specific age, disease and patient groups. The differences mainly are in mucosal adhesion of probiotic organism from different age groups and the influence of disease on mucosal adhesion of selected probiotics (Ouwehand *et al.*, 2002). The use of specially selected probiotics for particular subject groups may provide more specific health effects.

Alternative Applications

Probiotics are mainly used to influence the composition or activity of the intestinal microflora. However, any part of the body which harbors a normal microflora could be a potential target for specific probiotics to sustain in that region.

The oral cavity has a microflora that equals the intestinal microflora in complexity. Here too, some of the members of the normal microflora have a detrimental effect on the host which may cause dental caries or periodontal disease. Probiotics have many potential applications in the oral cavity. Yoghurt has been observed to reduce the colonization by *Streptococcus mutans*, the specific microorganism responsible for dental caries (Petti *et al.*, 2001). A specific probiotic *Lactobacillus* strain has been detected in saliva samples (Meurman *et al.*, 1994). Although there is a considerable potential for probiotic use in the oral cavity, more work needs to be done in this area.

The normal microflora of the urogenital tract is less complex than the microflora of the intestine and the oral cavity. However, more than 50 species are thought to colonize the urogenital tract for good health. Among these H_2O_2 producing *Lactobacilli* predominate (Lopez *et al.*, 1990). Disturbances in the *Lactobacillus* 287 flora are thought to be related to the risk for urinary tract infections. Some work has been done on the use of probiotics for urogenital tract infections. Selected *Lactobacillus* strains have been observed to reduce the recurrence of urinary tract infections (Reid *et al.*, 1992) and reduce the risk for vaginitis (Hilton *et al.*, 1992; Reid *et al.*, 2001).

Much work has also been done on the mechanisms of probiotic *Lactobacilli* on urinary tract infections; production of hydrogen peroxide and of biosurfactants appear to be important factors contributing to the efficacy of the probiotic strains for use in the urogenital tract (Reid, 2002). The probiotic *L. casei* shirota has been observed to reduce the recurrence of superficial bladder cancer (Aso *et al.*, 2002). These findings indicate that use of probiotics for the urogenital tract is a promising future area.

The skin has a normal microflora which is different depending on the site of the body. The most common genera found in the microflora of the skin are *Propionibacteria, Staphylococcus, Micrococcus, Corynebacterium* and the yeast *Malassezia*. Several species within these genera can be opportunistic pathogens. However, the potential use of probiotics for the skin has been considered little to none (Barefoot & Ratnam, 1998).

Also, the nasopharynx has a normal microflora, *Streptococcus pneumoniae* being frequently one of its normal members. *Lactobacilli* have been isolated from the upper respiratory tract. Their potential use as probiotics in there has only recently been considered and may have interesting applications (Cangemi de Gutierrez *et al*., 2000). Thus, there are many potential applications of probiotics which have received little attention but may provide significant health effects. Ishibashi and Yamazaki (2001) have discussed on the safety aspects of probiotics.

Jennifer and Sinderen (2014) have looked into the taxonomy of phages infecting lactic acid bacteria. Stanton (2003a) has studied the challenges ahead in the development of probiotic functional foods.

Vanden Nieuwboer *et al*. (2015) have qualitatively analyzed the innovation barriers in probiotic research and development. They have also discussed means to improve tech transfer cycle. Von Wright (2005) has explained the European approach to regulate the safety of probiotics. Zang *et al*. (2014) have studied the effect of multistrain probiotics on the growth performance, cecal microbial shedding and excreta odor contents in broilers. All these aspects are of great concern to the consumer today.

Multifunctional Genetically Improved Probiotic and Biomedical trend

The yeasts have a killer phenomenon which makes it a multicentric model for scientists, molecular biologists, virologists, phytopathologists, epidemiologists, industrial and medical microbiologists, mycologists, and pharmacologists. With a widespread appearance of this phenomenon among prokaryotic and eukaryotic pathogens it has brought a new interest in biology and product applications. The search for therapeutic opportunities by using yeast killer systems has conceptually opened new areasin the prevention and inhibition of fungal diseases by idiotypic network which is exploited by the immune system in the course of natural infections.

11
SACCHAROMYCES spp. AS PROBIOTICS

Today it has been understood that yeasts have great potentials as novel probiotics (Nayak, 2011). They have been found to be safe for human consumption in traditional fermented foods (Jakobsen and Narvhus 1996). Yeasts have a great physiological importance inside the gastrointestinal (GI) tract (Czerucka *et al.*, 2007; Gatesoupe, 2007). Jespersen (2003) has mentioned the role of consuming fermented foods and the health benefits attributed with it. Yeasts are known for prevention of table olive (Arroyo lopez *et al.*, 2012). Bonatsau *et al.* (2015) have shown multi-functional property of yeast as starters.

Beneficial physiological effects have been proved by *in vitro* and *in vivo* studies. Higher levels of antioxidants and lowering of blood cholesterol levels with the usage of probiotics have also been proved (Kumar *et al.*, 2012; Plessas *et al.*, 2012). During fermentation, yeasts produce many metabolites which have high antioxidant activity (Abbas, 2006). Yeasts come under GRAS category and help in high antioxidant activity, hypercholesterolaemia, an elevated level of cholesterol in the blood which is a major risk factor for cardiovascular diseases. These cover almost 45% of heart attacks (Kumar *et al.*, 2012). If serum cholesterol is reduced to 1% it helps in reducing heart disease mortality by almost 2% (Manson *et al.*, 1992). Reducing serum cholesterol with the use of Probiotics is receiving a lot of attention. This will help in preventing cardiovascular diseases. Psomas *et al.* (2003) have studied that yeast cells in the logarithmic phase have high ability to remove cholesterol. In Nigeria yeasts are characterized by a wide physiological diversity (Sanni and Lonner, 1993). The most important cereal-based traditional fermented food products are Burukutu (traditionally fermented beer), kunu-zaki (nonalcoholic fermented beverage) and ogi (fermented cereal gruel) in which yeasts commonly do the fermentation. Fermentation of traditional fermented cereal based foods cannot be predicted. In food fermentations yeasts occupy a very dominant place (Sanni and Lonner 1993; Akabanda *et al.*, 2013). Nutritional value and organoleptic properties of fermented foods has been attributed to the enzymes (Annan *et al.*, 2003; Hellstrom *et al.*, 2012). In a study done by Ogunremi *et al.* (2015) *C. tropicalis* BOM21, *P. kluyveri* LKC17, *I. orientalis* OSL11 and *P. kudriavzevii* OG32 and ROM11 produced enzymes of technological importance including protease, lipase and phytase. Esterase production was observed in *C. tropicalis* BOM21. It is well known that esterase and lipase improve the aromatic profile of fermented foods by increasing their free fatty acid content, which are precursors to the formation of different aromatic compounds. Phytase dephosphorylate phytate, an antinutrient factor present in cereals was studied by Raghavendra and Halami (2009). These enzymes have been reported for yeast in different organisms (Psomas *et al.*, 2001; Omemu *et al.*, 2007). Gotcheva *et al.* (2002) studied the tolerance to (2%) bile salts in the strains of *Trichosporon cutaneum*, *Candida rugosa* and *Candida lambica*. This is rare and has been reported for very few probiotic lactic acid bacteria. Agrawal *et al.* (2000) studied the flavour profile of idli batter prepared for defined microbial starter cultures and their beneficial uses. Fermentation technologies for smaller communities were studied by Rati *et al.* (2003). Gastric juice and pepsin are the two antimicrobial factors present in the stomach where as pancreatin and bile is present in the intestine. Psomas *et al.* (2001) have shown that many yeast strains showed satisfactory survival in gastric juice aspirated from human volunteers. Rajkowska and Kunicka-Styczynska (2010) have shown high tolerance to simulated conditions in the stomach and intestine with the strains of *S.cerevisiae*. Adherence ability to epithelial cells and to the mucosal surfaces is critical for probiotic selection (Duary *et al.,* 2011; Kechagia *et al.*, 2013). The property to adhere to the epithelial layer in yeast could be correlated with aggregation and also with the hydrophobic properties on the cell surface (Rosenberg *et al.*, 1980; Collado *et al.*, 2007).

Hydrophobicity was confirmed using organic solvents like n-hexadecane, toluene and octane. Strong adherence property was also observed in the strains of *W. anomalus*, *P. kudriavzevii* and *Kodamaea ohmeri* from broilers excreta (Garcða-Hernandez *et al.*, 2012). This is supported by a study by Sourabh *et al.* (2012), using n hexadecane, where some of their strains showed hydrophobicity above 50%. Adherence properties of yeast species have been supported by reports using several *in vitro* intestinal epithelial cell models at different levels (Kumura *et al.*, 2004; Chen and Xu 2010; Kourelis *et al.*, 2010). Makri *et al.* (2010) have studied the metabolic activities of the strains of *Y. lipolytica* grown on glycerol.

A very important property in yeasts is the activity against pathogenic microorganisms that can improve the shelf life and safety of fermented foods (Psani and Kotzekidou 2006). This has the competitive prevention of the colonization by pathogens to the intestine (Plessas *et al.*, 2012). According to Kourelis *et al.* (2010) and Perricone *et al.* (2014) yeasts do not produce antibacterial metabolites or have antagonistic activity against pathogens. In *in vitro* and *in vivo* studies only some yeast species have shown to lower the cholesterol level. However, this ability has been reported for several probiotic lactic acid bacteria (Kimoto *et al.*, 2002; Pan *et al.*, 2011). Yeasts strains that can remove cholesterol from culture medium by assimilation have been well worked out earlier (Psomas *et al.*, 2003; Chen *et al.*, 2013; Kourelis *et al.*, 2010). Cultures of *P. kudriavzevii*, BY10, *P. kudriavzevii* BY15, *Galactomyces* sp., BY1, *Pichia guilliermondii* BY31 have shown ability to assimilate cholesterol (Chen *et al.*, 2013).

There are number of products which are based on yeast fermentations. Brewer's yeast is the best characterized microorganism for food and beverage production. It is important to know the physiology, genetics and metabolism of this eukaryotic microorganism. There are many compounds produced by yeasts which are added to food after purification. Production of flavors and colors by yeasts also has a great potential. Generoso *et al.* (2010) and Gilliland *et al.* (2010) have shown the importance of yeast in protecting bacterial translocation and enhancing immunity.

The origin of fermented food can be traced back to 4000-3500 BC in Egypt. In Europe brewing was first developed in abbeys by the monks (Corran, 1975).

It was in 1680, when Antonie van Leeuwenhoek saw them under the microscope. It was Louis Pasteur who analyzed alcoholic fermentations quantitatively and stated that fermentation changes are associated with vital activity of yeasts. Also that glycerol and succinic acid were derived from the transformation of sugar during fermentation (Barnett, 2000). Characterizing microorganisms has become easier with novel techniques.

Many yeast strains are very important and are characterized by intrinsic genetic complexity. The yeast strains were found to be genetically diverse, prototrophic, homothallic and were either aneuploid, polyploid or alloploid. Liu *et al.* (2012) have shown simultaneous saccharification and microbial lipid fermentation of corn stover by oleaginous yeast *Trichosporon cutaneum*. Lopandic *et al.* (2006) have been able to identify yeasts which are associated with milk products. Odunfa and Oyewole (1998) have studied the microbiology of African fermented food. Szajewska and Mrukowicz (2005) studied the effect of *S. boulardii* in the prevention of antibiotic associated diarrhea. Tamang (2009) studied the diversity of yeast in fermented foods and beverages.

The major food products derived from yeast fermentations are beer, wine, other alcoholic beverages and bread. *S.cerevisae* has the ability to produce many metabolites that contribute for the attributes of flavor, aroma and taste. The strains should be thoroughly characterized. A measure of the overall antioxidant capacity of the food may provide more relevant biological informationcompared to that obtained by the measurement of individual components. According to Ogunremi *et al*. (2015) the overall antioxidant capacity of the cereal-based food increased after fermentation by *Pichia kudriavzevii* OG32. Similar results were found by Qian *et al*. (2012) where in their study they showed an increase in the antioxidant capacity of Pavlovalutheri (microalgae) after fermentation with Hansenula polymorpha (*Pichia angusta*). This could be due to the cell components of yeasts or metabolites with antioxidant activity. Oxygenated carotenoids, organicacids, glutathione, some uncharacterized proteins and cell wall β-glucan from yeasts have been characterized to have antioxidant properties (Abbas 2006; Balasubramanian and Ragunathan 2012). Siddiqui *et al.* (2012) have discussed the secondary metabolite biosynthesis in yeasts with synthetic biology tools.

Wine Production

Fermentation of grapes to wine is known to be challenging. With the use of defined starter cultures as inoculum it has become easier (Pretorius, 2000). Also the role of non-Sacc. yeasts are now being reassessed as it is possible to have a positive role in the product. Scientists are trying to add *S.cerevisae* in mixed starter cultures which is proving to be a very valuable tool (Ciani *et al.*, 2006). Sindhu and Khetarpaul (2003) have studied the effect on anti-nutrients and digestibility of starch and protein in food mixture.

It is important to know the probiotic effects, transcriptome, proteome and exo metabolome analysis in understanding different aspects of wine fermentations. Fermentation by yeasts and lactic acid bacteria have been studied by different workers (Annan *et al.*, 2003; Callejon *et al.*, 2010; Parkouda *et al.*, 2011; Sørensen *et al.*, 2011).

As the volatile compounds play a major role in imparting flavours to the product this aspect has been studied at large. The most abundant volatile compounds in the functional food are acids and esters accounting for 32.21 and 32.37%, respectively. The available information in the literature affirmed the flavor properties of some of the detected volatile compounds. Esters mainly determine the pleasant aromatic notes of fermented products, contributing to the flora and fruity odors (Chen and Xu 2010; Moreira *et al.*, 2011; Parkouda *et al.*, 2011). Flavor active acids detected in the fermented product include tetradecanoic acid, which has a creamy and cheesy flavor and 9, 12-octa de cadienoic acid with a faint fatty flavor (The Good Scent Company, TGSC). These compounds were reported in unfermented and fermented baobab seeds (Parkouda *et al.*, 2011). The proportion of higher alcohols was observed to be low in the fermented food (10.12%) and relatively low concentrations of higher alcohols contribute to fruity-like aromas for foods while at higher concentrations they contribute to the hot and irritating aromas, which are undesirable to the consumer (Saberi *et al.*, 2012). Benzyl alcohol is the largest proportion of alcohol in the fermented food. Benzyl alcohol has been reported in organic red wines fermented with *Saccharomyces cerevisiae* (Callejon *et al.*, 2010). It has sweet, floral, and fruity flavor with balsamic nuances (The Good Scent Company (TGSC, 1989).

The genetic complexity of brewer's yeasts makes transcriptomics more complex. DNA microarrays are used to map which map the conditions of high gravity fermentations (Piddocke *et al.*, 2011). Genes which are involved in stress responses and in amino acid metabolism have been identified. Combina *et al.* (2005) have studied the dynamics of indigenous yeast populations during spontaneous fermentation of wines. Fleet and Balia (2006) have explained the role of yeasts in foods and beverages. Psani *et al.* (2006) have studied the technological characteristics of yeast strains as starter adjuncts in olive fermentation.

References

Abbas CA.2006. Production of antioxidants, aromas, colours, flavours, and vitamins by yeasts. The yeast handbook: yeasts in food and beverages. Eds. Querol A and Fleet G H. Springer, Berlin, Heidelberg. 285-334.

Abdel Rahman H, Baraghit GA, Abu El-Ella AA, Omar SS, Abo Ammo FF, Kommona OF.2012. Physiological responses of sheep to diet supplementation with yeast culture. Egyptian J Sheep & Goat Sci. 7: 27-38.

Abdelbasset M and Djamila K. 2008. Antimicrobial activity of autochthonous lactic acid bacteria isolated from Algerian traditional fermented milk. RaïbAfr J Biotechnol. 7:2908-2914.

Abdel-Haleem WH, TinayAH E, Mustafa AI, Babiker EE. 2008. Effect of fermentation, malt-pretreatment and cooking on antinutritional factors and protein digestibility of sorghum cultivars. Pakistan J Nutr. 7: 335-341.

Abenavoli L, Petruzzellis C, Gasbarrini G and Gasbarrini A. 2008. Probiotics: which and when?" Digestive Dis. 26:175-182.

Abratt V R and Reid S J. 2010. Oxalate-degrading bacteria of the human gut as probiotics in the management of kidney stone disease. Adv Appl Microbiol. 72: 63-87. Academic Press.

Adhikari K, Mustapha A and Grun I U. 2003. Survival and metabolic activity of microencapsulated *Bifidobacterium longum* in stirred yogurt. J Fd Sci. 68: 275-280.

Adhikari K, Mustapha A, Grun I U and Fernando L. 2000. Viability of microencapsulated Bifidobacteria in yogurt during refrigerated storage. J Dairy Sci 83: 1946-1951.

Agerholm-Larsen L, Raben A, Haulrik N, Hansen AS, Manders M and Astrup A. 2000. Effect of 8 week intake of probiotic milk products on risk factors for cardiovascular diseases. Eur J Clin Nutr 54: 288-289.

Agostoni P1, Biondi-Zoccai GG, de Benedictis ML, Rigattieri S, Turri M, Anselmi M, Vassanelli C, Zardini P, Louvard Y, Akabanda H M et al., 2004. Radial versus femoral approach for percutaneous coronary diagnostic and interventional procedures; Systematic meta-overview and analysis of randomized trials. J Am Coll Cardiol. 44(2):349-56.

Agrawal R, Rati ER, Vijayendra SVN, Varadaraj MC, Prasad MS, Nand K. 2000. Flavour profile of idli batter prepared from defined microbial starter cultures. World J Microbiol Biotechnol. 16:687-690.

Agrawal Renu and Dharmesh S. 2012. An anti shigella dysenteriae bacteriocin from Pediococcus pentosaceous MTCC 5151 cheese isolate. Turk J Biol. 36:177-185.

Ahmed Z, Wang Y, Ahmad A, Tariq Khan S, Nisa M, Ahmad H, and Afreen A. 2013. Kefir and health: a contemporary perspective. Crit Rev Fd Sci Nutr. 53(5): 422-434.

Akabanda F, Owusu-KwartengJ, Tano-DebrahK, GloverR LK, Nielsen DS and Jespersen L. 2013. Taxonomic and molecular characterization of lactic acid bacteria and yeasts in nunu, a Ghanaian fermented milk product. Fd Microbiol. 34(2): 277-283.

Alm L. 1982. Effect of fermentation on lactose, glucose and galactose content in milk and suitability of fermented milk products for lactose-deficient individuals. J Dairy Sci.65: 346-352.

Almeida CC, Lorena SLS, Pavan CR et al., 2012. Beneficial effects of long-term consumption of a probiotic combination of *Lactobacillu scasei* Shirota and *Bifidobacterium breve* Yakult may persist after suspension of therapy in lactose in tolerant patients. Nutr Clin Prac. 27(2):247-251.

Alonso L, Cuesta E P and Gilliland SE. 2003. Production of free conjugated linoleic acid by *Lactobacillus acidophilus* and *Lactobacillus casei* of human intestinal origin. J Dairy Sci 86: 1941-1946.

Ambalam P, Dave JM, Nair BM, Vyas BR. 2011. *In vitro* mutagen binding and antimutagenic activity of human *Lactobacillus rhamnosus* 231. Anaerobe 17:217-222.

Ammor MS and Mayo B. 2007. Selection criteria for lactic acid bacteria to be used as functional starter cultures in dry sausage production: An update, Meat Sci. 76: 138-146.

Ammori BJ, Leeder PC, King RF, Barclay GR, Martin IG, Larvin M. et al. 1999. Early increase in intestinal permeability in patients with severe acute pancreatitis: correlation with endotoxemia, organ failure, and mortality. J Gastrointest Surg.3:252-62.

Anderson LW Ed, Krathwohl D R Ed., Airasian PW, Cruikshank KA, Mayer RE, Pintrich PR, Raths J and Wittrock MC. 2001. A taxonomy for learning, teaching, and assessing: A revision of Bloom's Taxonomy of Educational Objectives (Complete edition). New York: Longman and live lactic acid bacteria. FAO (UN).

Annan NT, Poll L, Sefa-DedeS, Plahar WA and Jakobsen M. 2003. Volatile compounds produced by *Saccharomyces Cerevisiae* and Candidakrusei in single starter culture fermentations of Ghanaian maize dough. J. Appl. Microbiol. 94:462-474.

Anonymous 2002. Guidelines for the Evaluation of Probiotics in Food. Report of a Joint FAO/WHO Working Group on Drafting Guidelines for the Evaluation of Probiotics in Food. London Ontario, Canada.

Anonymous 2010. Investigation Update: Multistate Outbreak of E. coli O157:H7 Infections Associated with Cheese. http://www.cdc.gov/ecoli/2010/cheese0157/index.html

Anonymous 2006. Ongoing multistate outbreak of Escherichiacoli serotype O157:H7 infections associated with consumption of fresh spinach-United States. Morb. Mortal. Wkly. Rep. 1045-1046.

Anonymous 2011. Investigation Announcement: Multistate Outbreak of *E.Coli* O157: H7 Infections Associated with Lebanon, Bologna.

Antonie Van Leeuwenhoek. 2002. Probiotics: an overview of beneficial effects. 82 (1-4):279 89.

Anukamk C, Osazuwae O, Semeneg I, Ehhigiagbe F, Brucea W and Reid G. 2006. Clinical study comparing probiotic *Lactobacillus* GR-1and RC-14 with metronidazole vaginal gel to treat symptomatic bacterial vaginosis. Microbes Infect. 8: 2772-2776.

Arerugi. 2006. Suppression of allergy development by habitual intake of fermented milk foods, evidence from an epidemiological study. 55(11):1394-9.

Argyri A, Zoumpopoulou G, Karatzas K A G, Tsakalidou E, Nychas GJE, Panagou EZ, Tassou C C. 2013. Selection of potential probiotic lactic acid bacteria from fermented olives by *in vitro* tests. Fd Microbiol. 33: 282-291.

Aronsson B, Barany P, Nord CE, et al. 1987. Clostridium difficile-associated diarrhea in uremic patients. Eur J Clin Microbiol. 6:352-356.

Arrigoni E, Marteau P, Briet F, Pochart P, Rambaud J C and Messing B. 1994.Tolerance and absorption of lactose from milk and yogurt during short-bowel syndrome in humans. Am J Clin Nutr. 60:926-929.

Arroyo-López FN, Querol A, Bautista-Gallego J and Garrido-Fernández A. 2008. Role of yeasts in table olive production. Inter J Fd Microbiol. 128:189-196.

Arroyo-Lopez FN, Romero-GilV, Bautista-Gallego J, Rodrõguez-Gomez F, Jimenez-Dõaz R, Garcõa-Garcõa P,Querol A and Garrido-Fernandez A. 2012. Yeasts in table olive processing: desirable or spoilage. Nutrition Rev. 65 (7): 316-328.

Aso Y and Akazan H. 1992. Prophylactic effect of a *Lactobacillus casei* preparation on the recurrence of superficial bladder cancer. Urol Int 49:125-129.

Aso Y,Akazan H, Kotake T, Tsukamoto T and Imai K. 1995. Preventive effect of a *Lactobacillus casei* preparation on the recurrence of superficial bladder cancer in a double-blind trial. Eur Urol. 27:104-109.

Aswathy RG, Ismail B, John RP and Nampoothiri KM. 2008. Evaluation of the probiotic characteristics of newly isolated lactic acid bacteria. Appl Biochem Biotechnol. 151 (23): 244-55.

Auffray Y, Gillot B, Lautier M, Thammavongs B and Boutibonnes P. 1989. Response of *Lactococcus lactis* to N-methyl-N-nitro-N-nitrosoguanidine: absence of adaptive response. Mutagenesis. 4: 280-282.

Ayad EHE, Verhenl A, de Jong C, Wonters J T M and Smith G. 1999. Flavour forming abilities and amino acid requirements of *Lactococcus lactis* isolated from artisanal and non dairy origin. Int Dairy J. 97: 25-735.

Baati LC, Fabre-Gea DA and Blanc PJ. 2000. Studyof the cryotolerance of *Lactobacillus acidophilus*: effect of culture and freezing conditions on the viability and cellular protein levels. Int J Fd Microbiol. 59: 241-247.

Badis A, Guetarni D, Moussa-Boudjemaa B, Henni DE and Kihal M. 2004. Identification and technological properties of lactic acid bacteria isolated from raw goat milk of four Algerian races. Fd Microbiol. 21: 579-588.

Balasubramanian K and Ragunathan R. 2012. Study of antioxidant and anticancer activity of natural sources. J Nat Prod Plant Resour. 2:192-197.

Balcázar JL, Vendrell D, de Blas I, Ruiz-Zarzuela I, Gironés O, Múzquiz JL. 2007. *In vitro* competitive adhesion and production of antagonistic compounds by lactic acid bacteria against fish pathogens. Veter Microbiol. 122 (3-4): 373-380.

Bamforth CW. 2005. Introduction Food, Fermentation and Microorganisms, Blackwell Publishing, UK, pp. XIV-XVI.

Bank MR, Kirksey A, West K and Giacoia G. 1985. Effect of storage time and temperature on folacin and vitamin C levels in term and preterm human milk. Am Jelin Nutr. 41: 235-242.

Bao Y, Zhang YC, Zhang Y, Liu Y, Wang SQ, Dong XM, Wang YY, Zhang HP. 2010. Screening of potential probiotic properties of *Lactobacillus fermentum* isolated from traditional dairy products. Food Control. 21(5): 695-701.

Barefoot SF and Ratnam P. 1998.Vaginales *Lactobacillus*-medikament. EP1011721A1

Barnett JA. 2000. A history of research on yeasts 2: Louis Pasteur and his contemporaries. 16(8):755-771

Baroja M, Lorea PV, Kirjavainen, S H and G Reid Bautista-Gallego *et al*. 2013. Anti-inflammatory effects of probiotic yogurt in inflammatory bowel disease patients. Clin Exp Immunol. 149(3): 470-479.

Barrangou R, Fremaux C, Deveau H, Richards M, Boyaval P, Moineau S, Romero DA, Horvath P. 2007. CRISPR Provides Acquired Resistance against Viruses in Prokaryotes. Science. 315(5819): 1709-1712.

Baruzzi F, Quintieri L, Morea M and Caputo L. 2011. Antimicrobial compounds produced by *Bacillus* spp. and applications in food science against microbial pathogens: communicating current research and technological advances.A. Méndez-Vilas (Ed).

Bautista-Gallego J, Arroyo-López FN, Kantsiou K, Jiménez Días R, Garrido Fernández A, Cocolin L. 2013. Screening of lactic acid bacteria isolated from fermented table olives with probiotic potential. Fd Res Int.50:135-142.
Bayless TM. 1981. Lactose malabsorption, milk intolerance, and symptom awareness in adults. In: Lactose digestion: clinical and nutritional implications. Paige DM, Bayless TM, eds. Baltimore: Johns Hopkins University Press: 117-23.
Beal C, Fonseca F and Corrieu G. 2001. Resistance to freezing and frozen storage of Streptococcus thermophilus is related to membrane fatty acid composition. J Dairy Sci. 84: 2347-2356.
Beasley S, Tuorila H and Saris PEJ. 2003. Fermented soymilk with monoculture of *Lactococcus lactis*. Int J Fd Microbiol. 81:159-162.
Berg G. 2009. Plant-microbe Interactions Promoting Plant Growth and Health: Perspectives for Controlled Use of Microorganisms in Agriculture. Appl Microbiol Biotech. 84:11-18.
Berg RD. 1996. The indigenous gastrointestinal microflora. Trends Microbiol. 4: 430-435.
Bergogne-Berezin E.2000.Treatment and prevention of antibiotic associated diarrhea Intern J Antimicrob Agents. 16(4): 521-526.
Besselink MG, van Santvoort HC, Buskens E, Boermeester MA, van Goor H, Timmerman HM, *et al.* 2008. Probiotic prophylaxis in predicted severe acute pancreatitis: a randomised, double-blind, placebo-controlled trial. Lancet 371: 651-659.
Betsi GI, Papadavid E, Falagas ME. 2008. Probiotics for the treatment or prevention of atopic dermatitis: a review of the evidence from randomized controlled trials. Am J Clin Dermatol.9 (2):93-103.
BgVV. 2000. Probiotische Mikroorganismen kulturen in Lebensmitteln. Abschlussbericht der Arbeitsgruppe —Probiotische Mikroorganismen in Lebensmitteln" am Bundesinstitut für gesundheitlichen Verbraucherschutz und Veterinärmedizin Berlin. In: Ernährungs-Umschau 47:191-195.
Black FT, Andersen PL, Ørskov F, Gaarslev K and Laulund S.1989. Prophylactic efficacy of lactobacilli on traveller's diarrhoea. Travellers Med. 8:1750-1753.
Blandino A,Al-Aseeri ME, Pandiella SS, Cantero D and Webb C. 2003. Cereal-based fermented foods and beverages. Fd Res Intern. 36: 527-543.
Bleichner G, Blehaut H, Mentec H and Moyse D. 1997. Saccharomyces boulardii prevents diarrhea in critically ill tube-fed patients. A multicenter, randomized, double-blind placebo-controlled trial. Intensive Care Med. 23:517-523.
Boasso A, Herbeuval JP, Hardy AW, et al. 2007. HIV inhibits CD4 (+) T-cell proliferation by inducing indoleamine 2, 3-dioxygenase in plasmacytoid dendritic cells. Blood.109: 3351-3359. ISSN: 0006-4971.
Bohnhoff N, Drake BL, Muller CP. 1954.Effect of streptomycin on susceptibility of the intestinaltract to experimental Salmonella infection. Bacteriol Proc. 56.
Boirivant M, Strober W. 2007. The mechanism of action of probiotics. Curr Opin Gastroenterol. 23:679-692.
Bonatsou S, Benítez A, Rodríguez Gomez F, Panagou E Z and Arroyo Lopez F N. 2015. Selection of yeasts with multifunctional features for application as starters in natural black table olive processing. Fd Microbiol. 46:66-73.
Borriello SP, Hammes WP, Holzapfel W, Marteau P, Schrezenmeir J, Vaara M, Valtonen V. 2003. Safety of probiotics that contain *Lactobacilli* or *Bifidobacteria*. Clin Infect Dis. 6(6): 775-780.
Bottone EJ. 2010. *Bacilluscereus*, a Volatile Human Pathogen. Clin Microbiol Rev. 23(2): 382-398.
Bourdichon F, Casaregola S, Farrokh C, Frisvad JC, Gerds ML, Hammes WP, Harnett J, Huys G, Laulund S, Ouwehand A, Powell IB, Prajapati JB, Seto Y, Ter Schure E, Van Boven A, Vankerckhoven V, Zgoda A, Tuijtelaars S, Hansen EB. 2012. Food fermentations: microorganisms with technological beneficial use. Int J Fd Microbiol. 154 (3): 87-97.

Boyle RJ, Bath-Hextall FJ, Leonardi BJ, Murrell DF and Tang M L. 2008. Probiotics for treating eczema. Cochrane Database Syst Rev. 4:135.
Braat H, Van Den Brande J, Van Tol E, Hommes D, Peppelenbosch M, Van Deventer S. 2004. *Lactobacillus rhamnosus* induces peripheral hyporesponsiveness in stimulated CD4$^+$ T cells via modulation of dendritic cell function. 1618-1625.
Brady LJ, Gallaher DD and Busta F. 2000. The role of probiotic cultures in the prevention of colon cancer. The J Nutri. 410S-414S.
Brassart D, Dannet-Hughes A, Neeser JR et al. 1995. Dairy bacterial strains with probiotic properties: Criteria for selection. IDF Nutrition Newsletter. 4: 29-32.
Bremer E and Kramer R. 2000. Coping with osmotic challenges: osmoregulation through accumulation and release of compatible solutes in bacteria. In: Storz G., Hengge-Aronis R. (Eds.), Bacterial Stress Responses, Chapter6, 79-97, ASM Press, Washington, D.C., 501 (ISBN 1-55581-192-2).
Briet F, Pochart P, Marteau P, Flourié B, Arrigoni E, Rambaud JC.1997. Improved clinical tolerance to chronic lactose ingestion in subjects with lactose intolerance: a placebo effect? Gut. 41:632-635.
Briggiler M M, Zacarías MF, Vinderola G, Reinheimer JA and QuiberoniA. 2014. Biological and probiotic characterization of spontaneous phage-resistant mutants of *Lactobacillus plantarum*. Intern Dairy J. 39(1).
Briggiler M, Quiberoni A. del L, Negro AC, Reinheimer J A,Alfano O M. 2011. Evaluation of the photocatalytic inactivation efficiency of dairy bacteriophages. Chem. Eng. J. 172: 987-993.
Brown MS, Goldstein JL. 1984. How LDL receptors influence cholesterol and atherosclerosis. Sci Am. 251(5):58-66.
Bruno FA and ShahNP. 2003. Viability of two freeze-dried strains of Bifidobacterium and of commercial preparations at various temperatures during prolonged storage. J Fd Sci. 68: 2336-2339.
Buckenhüskes HJ.1993. Selection criteria for lactic acid bacteria to be used as starter cultures for various food commodities. FEMS. Microbiol. Rev. 12: 253-272.
Bulletin of the International Federation. 2001. Bulletin of the international dairy federation.362/ 2001. Reviewed. Elad D.56 (3).
Bultman SJ. 2014. Emerging roles of the microbiome in cancer. Carcinogenesis. 35(2): 249-255.
Burnett LE, IkerdJ L and Burnett KG. 2006. Immune defense reduces respiratory fitness in Callinectes sapidus, the Atlantic blue crab. Biol Bull. 211: 50-57.
Burns AJ and Rowland IR. 2004. Antigenotoxicity of probiotics on fecal water-induced DNA damage in human colon adenocarcinoma cells. Mutat Res. 551: 233-243.
Buts JP, De KN and De RL. 1994. Saccharomycesboulardii enhances rat intestinal enzyme expression by endoluminal release of polyamines. Pediatr Res. 36: 522-527.
Caglar E, Topcuoglu N, Cildir S K, Sandalli N and Kulekci G. 2009. Oral colonization by *Lactobacillus reuteri* ATCC 55730 after exposure to probiotics. Int J Paediatr Dent. 19:377 81.
Caglar Y, Aksoy S, Ilican S, Caglar M. 2009. Crystalline structure and morphological properties of undoped and Sn doped ZnO thin films Superlattices Microstruct. 46: 469-475.
Callejon R M, Clavijo A, Ortigueira P, Troncoso AM, Paneque P and Morales ML. 2010. Volatile and sensory profile of organic red wines produced by different selected autochthonous and commercial Saccharomyces cerevisiae strains. Anal. Chimi. Acta 660:68-75.
Canadian Dairy Commission, 2011, Milk ingredients@cdc-ccl.gc.ca

Canducci F, Cremonini F, Armuzzi A.2002. Probiotics and *Helicobacter pylori* eradication. Dig Liver Dis. 34 Suppl 2:S81-83.

Cangemi de Gutierrez R, Santos de Araoz V, Nader-Macias M E. 2000. Effect of intranasal administration of *Lactobacillus* fermentum on the respiratory tract of mice. Biol Pharm Bull. 23:973-978.

Cannon JP, Lee TA, Bolanos JT, Danziger LH. 2005. Pathogenic relevance of *Lactobacillus*: a retrospective review of over 200 cases. Eur J Clin Microbiol Infect Dis. 24: 31-40.

Caplice E, Fitzgerald GF.1999. Food fermentation: role of microorganisms in food production and preservation. Int. J. Fd Microbiol. 50: 131-149.

Carr FJ, Chill D and Maida N. 2002. The lactic acid bacteria: A literature survey. Crit Rev Micrbiol 28: 281-370.

Carvalho AS, Silva J, Ho P, Teixeira P, Malcata FX and Gibbs P. 2003b. Protective effect of sorbitol and monosodium glutamate during storage of freeze-dried lactic acid bacteria. Lait. 83: 203-210.

Carvalho AS, Silva J, Ho P, Teixeira P, Malcata FX and Gibbs P. 2004. Relevant factors for the preparation of freeze-dried lactic acid bacteria. Int Dairy J. 14: 835-847.

Carvalho AS, SilvaJ, Ho P, Teixeira P, Malcata FX and Gibbs P. 2003a. Effect of different sugars added to the growth and drying medium upon thermotolerance and survival during storage of freeze-dried *Lactobacillus delbrueckii* spp., bulgaricus. Biotechnol Prog. 20: 248-254.

Cazaubiel M and Cazaubiel JM. 2010. Assessment of psychotropic-like properties of a probiotic formulation (Lactobacillushelveticus R0052 and *Bifidobacterium longum* R0175) in rats and human subjects. Brit J Nutr. 105:755-764.

Champagne C P and Gardner NJ.2005. Challenges in the addition of probiotic cultures to foods. Crit Rev Food Sci Nutr. 45: 61-84.

Champagne C, Mondou P, Raymond Fand Brochu E.1996. Effect of immobilization in alginate on the stability of freeze dried *Bifidobacterium longum*. Biosci Microflora.15: 9 15.

Champagne CF, Gardner N, Brochu E and Beaulieu Y.1991.The freeze drying of lactic acid bacteria. A rev. Canad. Institute of Fd Sci Technol J. 24: 118-28.

Champagne CP.2009. Some Technological Challenges in the Addition of Probiotic Bacteria to Foods. In: Charalampopoulos D, Rastall RA, editors. New York, Springer.761-804.

Chandramouli V, Kailasapathy K, Peiris P and Jones M. 2004. An improved method of microencapsulation and its evaluation to protect *Lactobacillus* spp. in simulated gastric conditions. J Microbial Methods. 57: 27-35.

Chapman C. M. C., Gibson G. R., Rowland I. 2014. Effects of single- and multi-strain probiotics on biofilm formation and in vitro adhesion to bladder cells by urinary tract pathogens. Anaerobe 27: 71-76.

Charalampopoulos D, Pandiella SS and Webb C. 2002a. Growth studies of potentially probiotic lactic acid bacteria in cereal based substrates. J App Microbiol. 92: 851-859.

Charalampopoulos D, Wang R, Pandiella SS and Webb C. 2002b. Application of cereals and cereal components in functional foods: a review. Int J Food Microbiol. 79: 131-141.

Charteris WP, Kelly PM, Morelli L and Collins JK. 1997. Selective detection, enumeration and identification of potentially probiotic *Lactobacillus* and *Bifidobacterium* species in mixed bacterial populations. Int J Fd Microbiol. 35:1-27.

Charteris WP, Kelly PM, Morelli L and Collins K. 1998. Antibiotic susceptibility of potential probiotic Lactobacillus species. J. Food Protect. 61:1636-1643.

Chavarri FJ, Paz MD and Neez MM.1988. Cryoprotective agents for frozen concentrated starter form non-bitter Streptococcus lactis strains, Biotechnol Lett. 10:10-16.

Chen L, Yang J, Yu J, Yao Z, Sun L, Shen Y, Jin Q. 2005. VFDB: a reference database for bacterial virulence factors. Nucleic Acids Res. 33:325-332.

Chen S and Xu Y. 2010. The influence of yeast strains on the volatile flavour compounds of Chinese rice wine. J Inst Brew. 116:190-196.
Chen SL, Wu M, Henderson JP, et al. 2013. Diversity and fitness of E. coli strains recovered from the intestinal and urinary tracts of women with recurrent urinary tract infections. Sci Transl Med.5 (184):184ra60.
Chen YS, Wu HC, Wong CM *et al*. 2013. Isolation and characterization of lactic acid bacteria from pobuzini (fermented Cumming cordia) a traditional fermented food in Taiwan. Folia Microbiologia. 58 (2): 103-109.
Chin LG and Busta F F. 2000. The role of probiotic cultures in the prevention of colon cancer. The J Nutri. 410S-414.
Chitme HR, Ramesh C, Sadhna K. 2004. Study of Antidiarrhoeal activity of Calatropsisgigantean in experimental animals. JPharmacol Pharm Sci. 7:70-75.
Chou C and Hou J. 2000. Growth of Bifidobacteria in soymilk and their survival in the fermented soymilk drink during storage. Inter J Fd Microbiol. 56: 113-121.
Chouraqui JP, Grathwohl D, Labaune JM, et al. 2008. Assessment of the safety, tolerance, and protective effect against diarrhea of infant formulas containing mixtures of probiotics or probiotics and prebiotics in a randomized controlled trial. Am J Clin Nutr. 87(5):1365-1373.
Christophe M, Kuczkowska K, Langella P, Eijsink VG, Mathiesen G, Chatel JM.2015. Surface display of an anti-DEC-205 single chain Fv fragment in *Lactobacillus plantarum* increases internalization and plasmid transfer to dendritic cells *in vitro* and *in vivo*. Microb Cell Fact.14:95.
Chuayana Jr EL, Ponce CV, Rivera MRB and Cabrera EC. 2003. Antimicrobial activity of probiotics from milk products. Phil JMicrobiol Infect Dis. 32: 71-74.
Ciani M, Beco L and Comitini F. 2006. Fermentation behavior and metabolic interactions of multi starter wine yeast fermentations. Int J Fd Microbiol. 108: 239-45.
Clarke G, O'Mahony S M, Hennessy A A, Ross P, Stanton C, Cryan J F and Dinan T G. 2009. Chain reactions: early-life stress alters the metabolic profile of plasma polyunsaturated fatty acids in adulthood. Behav. Brain Res. 205: 319-321.
Collado MC, Hernandez M, Sanz Y. 2005. Production of bacteriocin-like inhibitory compounds by human fecal *Bifidobacterium strains* J Food Prot 68: 1034-1040.
Collado MC, Meriluoto J and Salminen S. 2007. Measurement of aggregation properties between probiotics and pathogens: *In vitro* evaluation of different methods. JMicrobiol Methods. 71: 71-74.
Combina M, Elia A, Mercado L, Catania C, Ganga A and Martinez C. 2005. Dynamics of indigenous yeast populations during spontaneous fermentation of wines from Mendoza, Argentina. Int. J. Fd. Microbiol. 99:237-243.
Comelli EM, Guggenheim B, Stingele F and Neeser JR.2002. Selection of dairy bacterialstrains as probiotics for oral health. Eur. J. Oral Sci.110 (3):218-24.
Conway P L, Gorbach S L and Goldin B R. 1987. Survival of lactic acid bacteria in the human stomach and adhesion to intestinal cells. J. Dairy Sci. 70:1-12.
Conway PL. 1995. Microbial ecology of the human large intestine. In: Human colonic bacteria: Role in nutrition, physiology and pathology.CRC press-Taylor and Francis Group. Eds. Gibson GR, Macfarlane GT. London, UK. 1-24.
Corcoran C, Malaspina D, Hercher L. 2005. Prodromal interventions for schizophrenia vulnerability: the risks of being —at risk. Schizophr Res.73 (2-3):173-184.
Corran HS.1975.A history of brewing, David and Charles Publishers, Vermont, Canada.
Corsetti A, Gobbetti M, Rossi J and Damiani P. 1998. Antimould activity of sourdough lactic acid bacteria: identification of a mixture of organic acids produced by *L.sanfranscisco* CB1. Appl Micro Biotech. 50: 253-256.

CRDF. California Dairy Research Foundation. 2015. Products with Probiotics.us.probiotics.org.

Cremonini F, DiCaro S and Nista EC.2002. Meta-analysis: the effect of probiotic administration on antibiotic-associated diarrhoea.Aliment Pharmacol Ther. 16(8):1461-1467.

Cromwell GL. 2002. Why and how antibiotics are used in swine production. IN: L.B. Schook, ed. Animal Biotechnology. Marcel Dekker, Monticello, New York. 13(1): 7-27.

Crooks N H, Snaith C, Webster D, Gao F and Hawkey P. 2012. Clinical review: Probiotics in critical care. Crit Care. 16(6): 237.

Crowe J H, Crowe L M, Carpenter AS, Rudolph AS, Aurell-Winstrom C, Spargo B J and Anchordoguy YI. 1988. Interaction of sugars with membranes. Biochimica Biophysica Acta 947: 367-384.

Crowe L M and Crowe J H1988. Trehalose and dry dipalmitoyl phosphatidylcholine revisited. Biochim Biophys Acta. 946:193-201.

Cummings J H, Christie S and Cole T J 2001. A study of fructo oligosaccharides in the prevention of travellers diarrhea. Alimentary Pharmacology Therapeutics.15:1139- 1145

Czerucka D, Piche T and Rampal P. 2007. Review article: yeast as probiotics- *Saccharomyces boulardii*. Alim Pharma Therap. 26: 767-778.

D'Aimmo MR, Mattarelli P, Biavati, B, Carlsson NG and Andlid T. 2012. The potential of Bifidobacteria as a source of natural folate. J Appl Microbiol. 112: 975-984.

Damaskos and Kolios. 2008. Probiotics and prebiotics in inflammatory bowel disease. Br J Clin Pharmacol. 65 (4):453-67.

Danfeng Song, Salam Ibrahim and Saeed Hayek. 2012. Immunology Microbiology and Probiotics, book edited by Everlon Cid Rigobelo, ISBN 978-953-51-0776-7, and Published: October 3, under CC BY 3.0 license. © The Author(s).

Dani C, Biadaioli R, Bertini G, Martelli E, Rubaltelli FF. 2002. Probiotics feeding in prevention of urinary tract infection, bacterial sepsis and necrotizing enterocolitis in preterm infants. A prospective double-blind study. Biol Neonate. 82:103-108.

Daniells S. 2013. *L. rhamnosus* probiotic shows long-lasting anti-eczema benefits for kids: RCT. Daily supplements containing the probiotic *Lactobacillus rhamnosus* HN001 strain may reduce the incidence of eczema and skin sensitivity in children, according to data from a double-blind randomized placebo-controlled trial.http://www.nutraingredients-usa.com/Research/ *L.rhamnosus*-probiotic-shows-long-lasting-anti-eczema-benefits-for-kids-RCT.

Das RR, Singh M, Shafiq N. 2010. Probiotics in treatment of allergic rhinitis.World Allergy Organ J. 3:239-244.

Dave RI, Shah NP. 1998. Ingredient supplementation effects on viability of probiotic bacteria in yoghurt. Dairy Sci. 81:2804-2816.

De simone R, Moran J, Schein SJ, Mishkin M.1993. A role for thecorpus callosum in the visual area V4 of the macaque. VisNeurosci 10:159-171.

De Smet I, De Boever P, Verstraete W.1998 Cholesterol lowering in pigs through enhanced bacterial bile salt hydrolase activity.Br J Nutr 79: 185-194.

De Smet I, Van Hoorde L, De Sayer N, Vande Woestyne M,Verstraete W.1994. Invitro study of bile salt hydrolase (BSH) activity of BSH isogenic *Lactobacillus plantarum* 80 strains and estimation of cholesterol lowering through enhanced BSHactivity. Microb Ecol Health D. 7: 315-329.

De Smet I, Van Hoorde L, Woestyne MV, Christiaens H, and Verstraete W. 1995. Significance of bile salt hydrolase activity of lactobacilli. J Appl Bacteriol. 79: 292-301.

De Vrese M, Winkler P, Rautenberg P, HarderT, Noah C, Laue C, Ott S, Hampe J, Schreiber S, Heller K and Schrezenmeir J. 2005. Effect of *Lactobacillus gasseri* PA 16/8, *Bifidobacterium longum* SP 07/3, *B. bifidum* MF 20/5 on common cold episodes: A doubleblind, randomized, controlled trial. Clin Nutr. 24(4):481-491.

De Vrese M, Keller B, Barth CA. 1992. Enhancement of intestinal hydrolysis of lactose by microbial β-galactosidase (EC 3.2.1.23) of kefir. Br J Nutr. 67:67-75.

De Vrese M, Suhr M, Barth CA.1995. Affinitäts chromatographische Differenzierung zwischen intestinaler und mikrobieller β-Galaktosidase im Darm der Ratte. (Differentiation of intestinal from bacterial β-galactosidase in the small intestine of rats by affinity chromatography.) Zeitschrift für Ernährungswissenschaft.; 34:40A (abstr; in German).

De Vuyst L, de Vin F, Vaningelgem F, Degeest B.2001. Recent development in the biodsynthesis and applications of heteropolysaccharides from lactic acid bacteria. Int. Dairy J. 11. 687- 707

De Zwart LL, Meerman J HN, Commandeur J NM, Vermeulen N PE.1999. Biomarkers of free radical damage: Applications in experimental animals and in humans. Free Radical Biology and Medicine. 26 (1-2):202-226.

Deeth HC and Tamime AY. 1981. Yogurt, nutritive and therapeutic aspects. J Fd Prot. 44: 78-86.

Deibel RH and Niven CF. 1960. Comparative study of Gaffkya homari, Aerococcus viridans, tetrad forming cocci from meat curing brines and the genus Pediococcus. J. Bact. 79: 175.

Del Re B, Sgorbati B, Miglioli M and Palenzona D. 2000. Adhesion, autoaggregation and hydrophobicity of 13 strains of *Bifidobacterium longum*. Lett Appl Microbiol. 31: 438- 442.

Delcenserie V, Martel D, Lamoureux M, Amio J, Boutin Y and Roy D. 2008.Curr. Issues Mol. Biol. 10: 37-54. Online journal at http://www.cimb.org. Immunomodulatory Effects of Probiotics in the Intestinal Tract.

Deng J, Cheng W and Yang G. 2011. A novel antioxidant activity index (AAU) for natural products using the DPPH assay. Food Chemistry. 125: 1430-1435.

Deshmukh DS, Zanjad PN, Pawar VD, Machewad GM. 2009. Studies on the use of acidified and cultured whey as coagulant in the manufacture of paneer. Int J Dairy Technol. 62(2): 174- 181.

Deshpande G, Rao S and Patole S.2007. Probiotics for prevention of necrotising enterocolitis in preterm neonates with very low birthweight: A systematic review of randomised controlled trials. Lancet. 369:1614-20.

Devery R, Miller A and Stanton C. 2001. Conjugated linoleic acid and oxidative behavior in cancer cells. Biochem Soci Trans. 9: 341-344.

Dias A C F, Andreote F D, Hannula SE, Andreote FD, Silva M de CP, Salles JF, Boer W de, vanVeen J, van Elsas JD. 2013. Different selective effects on rhizosphere bacteria exerted by genetically modified versus conventional potato lines. PLOS ONE. www.plosone.org.8 (7): e67948.

Diebel RH, Wilson GD and Niven CF.1961. Microbiology of meat curing IV. A lyophilized Pediococcus cerevisiae starter culture for fermented sausage. Appl Microbiol. 9: 239-243.

Dinesh Kumar and Renu Agrawal 2008. Preparation of probiotic fermented milk using a native isolate of Pediococcus pentosaceous MTCC 5151. Res J Biotechnol. 3(4): 28-31.

Ding WK and Shah NP. 2009. Effect of various encapsulating materials on the stability of probiotic bacteria. J Fd Sci. 74(2): M100-7. Change shah 2009 in text

Donkor ON, Nilmini SLI, Stolic P, Vasiljevic T, Shah NP. 2007. Survival and activity of selected probiotic organisms in set-type yoghurt during cold storage. Int Dairy J. 17:657- 665.

Donohue D C and Salminen S.1996. Safety assessment of probiotic bacteria. Asia Pac J Clin Nutr. 5:25-28.

Doron SI, Hibberd PL, Gorbach SL. 2008. Probiotics for prevention of antibiotic- associated diarrhea. J Clin Gastroenterol. 42 Suppl 2: 58-63.

Douglas LC, Sanders ME.2008. Probiotics and prebiotics in dietetics practice. Am Diet Assoc. 108(3):510-21.

Drake RE, O'Neal EL, Wallach MAA. 2008. Systematic review of psychosocial research on psychosocial interventions for people with co-occurring severe mental and substance use disorders. JSubs Abuse Treat. 34:123-138.

Drici-Cachon Z, Cavin JF. Divies C.1996.Effect of pH and age of culture on cellular fatty acid composition of Leuconostocoenos. Lett Appl Microbiol. 22:331-334.

Duary RK, Rajput Y S, Batish V K and Grover S. 2011. Assessing the adhesion of putative indigenous probiotic lactobacilli to human colonic epithelial cells. Ind J Med Res. 134(5): 664-671.

Duary RK, Rajput YS, Batish VK, Grover S. 2011. Assessing the adhesion of putative indigenous probiotic lactobacilli to human colonic epithelial cells.Ind J Med Res. 134(5):664 71.

Duc Le H, Hong HA, Uyen NQ, Cutting SM.Vaccine. 2004. Intracellular fate and immunogenicity of B. subtilis spores.7, 22(15-16):1873-85.

Duc Le H, Hong HA, Barbosa TM, Adriano OH and Simon MC. 2004. Characterization of Bacillus Probiotics Available for Human Use. Appl Environ Microbiol.70 (4): 2161-2171.

Dugas B, Mercenier A, Lenoir-Wijnkoop I, Arnaud C, Dugas N and Postaire E .1999. Immunity and probiotics. Immunol Today. 20: 387-390.

Duncan SH, Flint HJ.2013. Probiotics and prebiotics and health in ageing populations. Maturitas.75: 44-50.

Dunne C, O'Mahony L, Murphy L, Thornton G, Morrissey D, O'Halloran S, Feeney M, Flynn S, Fitzgerald G, Daly C, Kiely B, C O'Sullivan G, Shanahan F and Collins JK. 2001. *In vitro* selection criteria for probiotic bacteria of human origin: Correlation with *in vivo* findings. Am J Clin Nutr.73:386S-392S.

Duwat P, Ehrlich S D and Gruss A. 1992. A general method for cloning rec A genes of gram-positive bacteria by polymerasechain reaction. J Bacteriol. 174: 5171-5175.

Dziuba B and Dziuba M. 2014. Milk proteins-derived bioactive peptides in dairy products: molecular, biological and methodological aspects. Acta Sci Pol Technol Aliment. 13(1): 5- 25.

Elmer GW, Surawicz CM, McFarland LV. 1996. Biotherapeutic agents. A neglected modality for the treatment and prevention of selected intestinal and vaginal infections. JAMA. 275: 870-6.

Enas EA. 2005. How to beat the heart disease epidemic among South Asians: A prevention and management guide for Asian Indians and their doctors. Downers Grove: Advanced Heart Lipid Clinic. (Book)

Enas GG. 1998. The Statistics Organization of the Future within the Pharmaceutical Industry. Pharma Biostatistics Subsection, Biostatistics and Clinical Data Management Annual Workshop

Endo Y, Kamisada S, Fujimoto K and Saito T. 2006. Trans fatty acids promote the growth of some Lactobacillus strains. J Gen Appl Microbiol. 52: 29-35.

Erdogrul O and Erbilir F.2006. Isolation and characterization of Lactobacillusbulgaricus and Lactobacilluscasei from various foods. Turk J. Biol. 30: 39-44.

Escherichia coli O78:K80 in poultry. Veter Microbiol. 79: 133 142.

Fabio M, FabianoV, Mameli Cand Zuccotti GV. 2012. Pharmaceuticals (Basel). Probiotics and Atopic Dermatitis in Children. 5(7): 727-744.

Famularo G, De Simone C, Pandey V, Sahu AR and Minisola G. 2005. Probiotic *Lactobacilli*: an innovative tool to correct the malabsorption syndrome of vegetarians.1132-5.

FAO/ WHO, 2001. Evaluation of health and nutritional properties of powdermilk.

FAO/ WHO. 2002a. Drafting Guidelines for the Evaluation of Probiotics in Food London Ontario, Canada.

FAO/WHO. 2002b. Guidelines for the evaluation of probiotics in food. Report of a joint FAO/ WHO working group on drafting guidelines for the evaluation of probiotics in food, London, Ontario, Canada.1-11.

FAO/WHO.1973. Bull World Health Organ.1979.57 (1):65-79.PMCID: PMC2395752. Protein and energy requirements: a joint FAO/WHO Memorandum.

Feleszko W, Jaworska J, Rha RD, Steinhausen S, Avagyan A, Jaudszus A, Ahrens B, Groneberg DA, Wahn U, Hamelmann E. 2007. Probiotic-induced suppression of allergic sensitization and airway inflammation is associated with an increase of T regulatory-dependent mechanisms in a murine model of asthma. Clin. Exp. Allergy 37 :498-505.

Femke L, Nijmeijer R M, Sandström PA,Trulsson LM, Magnusson KE, Timmerman HM, van Minnen L P, Rijkers G T, Gooszen H G, Akkermans LMA, and Söderholm JD.2009. Probiotics prevent intestinal barrier dysfunction in acute pancreatitis in rats via induction of ileal mucosal glutathione biosynthesis. PLOS ONE. 4(2): e4512.

Ferguson LR.1999. Natural and man-mademutagens and carcinogens in the diet. Introduction to special issue of mutation research. Mutat. Res. 443: 1 10.

Fernandes CF, Shahani KM and Amer MA. 1987. Therapeutic role of dietary *lactobacilli* and *lactobacilli* fermented dairy products. FEMS Microbiol Rev. 46: 343-356.

Fernandes CF, Shahani KM. 1990. Anticarcinogenic and immunological properties of dietary *Lactobacilli*. J. Food Prot.53:704-710.

Filippo C, Filippo C, Di Caro S, Santarelli L, Armuzzi A, Gasbarrini G, Gasbarrini A. 2001. Helicobacterpylori treatment: a role for Probiotics. Dig. Dis. 19:144-147.

Fleet GH and Balia R.2006. In Yeasts in Food and Beverages; Querol, A., Fleet, G.H., Eds.; Springer Verlag: Berlin, Heidelberg, Germany. 2: Chap.12.381-398.

Fleming HP, Mcfeeters RF, Thompson RL and Sanders DC. 1973. Storage stability of vegetables fermented with pH control. J Fd Sci.48: 975-981.

Folster-Holst R, Muller F, Schnopp N, Abeck D, Kreiselmaier I,et al. 2006. Prospective, randomized controlled trial on *Lactobacillus rhamnosus* in infants with moderate to severe atopic dermatitis. Br J Dermatol.155 (6):1256 -1261.

Fonseca F, Beal C and Corrieu G. 2000. Method for quantifying the loss of acidification activity of lacticacid starters during freezing and frozen storage. J. Dairy Res. 67:83-90.

Fooks LJ, Fuller R and Gibson GR.1999. Prebiotics, probiotics and human gut microbiology. Int. Dairy J. 9:53-61.

Foschino R, Perrone F, Galli A. 1995. Characterization of two virulent *Lactobacillus fermentum* bacteriophages isolated from sour dough. J. Appl. Microbiol. 79: 677-683.

Franceschi C, Capri M, Monti D, Giunta S, Olivieri F, Sevini F, Panourgia MP, Invidia L,Celani L,Scurti M,Cevenini E,Castellani GC, Salvioli S. 2007. Inflammaging and anti inflammaging: a systemic perspective on aging and longevity emerged from studies in humans. Mech Ageing Dev.128:92-105. Check in text

Franceschi C.2007. Inflammaging as a major characteristic of old people: can it be prevented or cured? Nutr Rev.65:S173-S176.

Franciosi E, Settanni L, Cavazza A, Poznanski E.2009.Biodiversity and technological potential of wild lactic acid bacteria from raw cows' milk. Int. Dairy J. 19(1): 3-11.

Franz CMAP, Huch M, Mathara JM, Abriouel H, Benomar N, Reid G, et al. 2014. African fermented foods and probiotics. Intern J Fd Microbiol. 190C: 84-96.

Frederick SA and Fridovich I.1981. Manganese and Defenses against Oxygen Toxicity in *Lactobacillus plantarum*. J Bacteriol. 145(1): 442-451.

Frolich-Wyder MT, Bachmann HP, Casey MG. 2002. Interactions between propionibacteria and starter/nonstarter lactic acid bacteria in Swiss-type cheese. Lait. 82: 1-15.

Frøyland L, Bentsen H, Graff IE, Myhrstad M, Paulsen JE, Retterstøl K, et al. 2011. Evaluation of Negative and Positive Health Effects of N-3 Fatty Acids as Constituents of Food Supplements and Fortified Foods. Opinion of the Steering Committee of the Norwegian Scientific Committee for Food Safety. Norwegian Scientific Committee for Food Safety (VKM): Oslo, Norway.

Fukushima M and Nakano M. 1995. The effect of a probiotic on faecal and liver lipid classes in rats. Brit J Nutr.73: 701-710.

Fuller R and Perdigon G. 2000. Probiotics-3. Immunomodulation by the gut microflora and probiotics. Kluver Academic Publishers.

Fuller R. 1989. Probiotics in man and animals. J Appl Bacteriol. 66(5):365-78.

Fuster V and Kelly B B. 2010. Promoting Cardiovascular Health in the Developing World. A Critical Challenge to Achieve Global HealthInstitute of Medicine (US) Committee on Preventing the Global Epidemic of Cardiovascular Disease: Meeting the Challenges in Developing Countries. Ed. Washington (DC): National Acad Press (US).ISBN-13: 978-0 309-14774-3ISBN-10: 0-309-14774-3.

Gabrial D, Sait SM, Hodgson A, Schmutz U, Kunin WE, Benton TG. 2010. Scale matters. The impact of organic farming on biodiversity at different spatial scales. Ecol Lett. 13(7): 858-869.

Gabriella C and Simon M. 2002. Cutting Bacillus Probiotics: Spore Germination in the Gastrointestinal Tract. Appl Environ Microbiol. 68(5): 2344-2352.

Gan BS, Kim J, Reid G Cadieux P and Howard J C.2002. *Lactobacillus fermentum* RC-14 Inhibits Staphylococcusaureus Infection of Surgical Implants in Rats. J Infect Dis. 185 (9): 1369-1.

García-Hernandez Y, Rodrðguez Z, Brandao LR, Rosa CA, Nicoli JR, Iglesias AE, Perez-Sanchez T, Salabarrða RB. et al. 2012. Identification and in-vitro screening of avian yeasts for use as probiotic. Res Vet Sci. 93: 798-802.

Garcia-Ruiaz A, Gonzalez de Llano D, Esteban F A, Requena T, Bartolome B and Moreno A M V. 2014. Assessment of probiotic properties in lactic acid bacteria isolated from wine. Fd Microbiol. 44:220-225.

Garrity, G.M., Boone, D.R. and Castenholz, R.W. (eds., 2001). Bergey's Manual of Systematic Bacteriology, 2nd ed., vol. 1, Springer-Verlag, New York, NY.

Gatesoupe FJ. 2007. Live yeasts in the gut: natural occurrence, dietary introduction, andtheir effects on fish health and development. Aquaculture 267: 20-30.

Gaurner F and Malagelada JR. 2003. Gut flora in health and disease.Lancet. 8;361(9356):512 9.

Gayathri Krishnan and Renu Agrawal 2012. Antioxidant activity and fatty acid profile of fermented milk prepared by Pediococcuspentosaceus. JFd SciTechnol.

Ge Z, White DA, Whary M T and Fox JG. 2001. Fluorogenic PCR-Based quantitative detection of a murine pathogen Helicobacterhepaticus. JClin Microbiol. 39: 2598-2602.

Generoso SV, Viana M, Santos R, Martins FS, Machado JA, Arantes RM. et al. 2010. *Saccharomyces cerevisiae* strain UFMG 905 protects against bacterial translocation preserves gut barrier integrity and stimulates the immune system in a murine intestinal obstruction model. Arch Microbiol.192:477-84.

Ghelardi EF, Celandroni S, Salvetti SA, Gueye A, Lupetti S, Senesi. 2015. Survival and persistence of *Bacillus clausii* in the human gastrointestinal tract following oral administration as spore-based probiotic formulation. J App. Micro. 119 (2): 552-559.

Giaouris E,Chapot-Chartier M, Briandet R. 2009. Surface physicochemical analysis of natural *Lactococcus lactis* strains reveals the existence of hydrophobic and low charged strains with altered adhesive properties. Int J Fd Microbiol. 131: 2-9.

Gilliland S E and Walker D K. 1989. Factors to consider when selecting a culture of *Lactobacillus acidophilus* as a dietary adjunct to produce a hypocholesteremic effect in humans. J Dairy Sci.73: 905-911.

Gilliland SE and Kim H.S.1983. Influence of Yogurt Containing Live Starter Culture on Lactose Utilization in Humans. Animal Sci Res Rep. 113-116.

Gilliland SE and Kim HS. 1984. Effect of viable starter culture bacteria in yogurt on lactose utilization in humans. J Dairy Sci.67:1-6.

Gilliland SE, Nelson CR and Maxwell C.1985. Assimilation of cholesterol by *Lactobacillus acidophilus*. Appl Environ Microbiol. 49(2): 377-381.

Gilliland SE, Staley TE and Bush LJ.1984b. Importance of bile tolerance of *Lactobacillus acidophilus* used as a dietary adjunct. J Dairy Sci. 67: 3045-3051.

Gilliland SV, Viana M, Santos R, Martins FS, Machado JA, Arantes RM. et al. 2010. *Saccharomyces cerevisiae* strain UFMG 905 protects against bacterial translocation preserves gut barrier integrity and stimulates the immune system in a murine intestinal obstruction model. Arch Microbiol.192:477-84.

Giovannini M, Agostoni C, Riva E, Salvini F, Ruscitto A, Zuccotti GV, et al. 2007. A randomized prospective double blind controlled trial on effects of long-term consumption of fermented milk containing *Lactobacilluscasei* in pre-school children with allergic asthma and/or rhinitis.Pediatr Res. 62 : 215-220.

Giraffa G. 1995. Enterococcal bacteriocins: theirpotential as anti-Listeria factors in dairytechnology. Fd Microbiol. 12:291-299.

Girigowda K and Mulimani VH. 2006. Hydrolysis of galacto- oligosaccharides in soy milk by K-carrageenan entrapped alpha-galactosidase from Aspergillusoryzae. World J Microbiol. Biotechnol. 22: 437-442.

Gismondo MR, Drago L. and Lombardi A. 1999. Review of probiotics available to modify gastrointestinal flora. Int J Antimicrobial Agents.12:287-292.

Giuliana Mastropietro, Inés Tiscornia, Karen Perelmuter, Soledad Astrada, and Mariela Bollati-Fogolín. 2015. Mediators of Inflammation. HT-29 and Caco-2 Reporter Cell Lines for Functional Studies of Nuclear Factor Kappa B Activation. ID 860534, 13 pageshttp://dx.doi.org/10.1155/2015/860534.

Giulio B De, Orlando P, Barba G, Coppola R, Rosa M De, De Prisco P P and Nazzaro F.2005. Use of Alginate and Cryo-Protective Sugars to Improve the Viability of Lactic Acid Bacteria after Freezing and Freeze-Drying.World J Microbiol Biotechnol. 21(5):739-746.

Gobbetti M, CagnoR Di and Angelis M De. 2010. Functional microorganisms for functional food quality. Crit. Rev. Fd Sci. Nutr. 50:716-727.

Godward G and Kailasapathy K. 2003. Viability and survival of free, encapsulated and co encapsulated probiotic bacteria in ice cream. Milchwissenschaft. 58: 161-164.

Goldberg I and Eschar L. 1977. Stability of lactic acid bacteria to freezing as related to their fatty acid composition. Appl Envi Micro. 33: 489-496.

Goldin B and Gorbach S.1980.Effect of Lactobacillusacidophilus dietary supplements on 1,2-dimethylhydrazine dihydrochloride-induced intestinal cancer in rats. JNatl Cancer Inst. 64: 263-265.

Goldin B R and Gorbach SL. 1976. The relationship betweendiet and rat fecal bacterial enzymes implicated in colon cancer.J Natl Cancer Inst. 57:371-377.

Goldin B, Gorbach SL and Chang TW. 1987. Successful treatment of relapsing *Clostridium difficile* colitis with *Lactobacillus* GG. Lancet. 1519.

Goldin BR and Gorbach SL. 1992. Probiotics for humans. In: Probiotics, Scientific Basis (Ed: Fuller, R.) Chapman and Hall, London, 355-376.

Goldin BR and Gorbach S L.1984. The effect of milk and lactobacillus feeding on human intestinal bacterial enzyme activity. Am J Clin Nutr. 39(5):756-761.

Goldin BR, Gualtien LJ and Moore RP.1996. The effect of Lactobacillus GG on the initiation and promotion of DMH-induced intestinal tumors in the rat. Nutr Cancer 25: 197-204.

Goldin BR, Swenson L, Dwyer J, Sexton M and Gorbach S. 1980. Effect of diet and *Lactobacillus acidophilus* supplements on human fecal bacterial enzymes. JNatl Cancer Inst. 64L: 225-261.

Gollin G, Marks C and Marks H.1993. Intestinal fatty acid binding protein in serum and urine reflects early ischemic injury to the small bowel. Surgery.113:545-551.

Gollop N, Zakin V, Weinberg Z G, Gonzalez et al. 2005. Antibacterial activity of lactic acid bacteria included in inoculants for silage and in silages treated with these inoculants. 98(3):662-666.

González B, Arca P, Mayo B and Suarez JE.1994.Detection, purification, and partial characterization of plantaricin C, a bacteriocin produced by a *Lactobacillus plantarum* strain of dairy origin. Appl Environ Microbiol. 60:2158-2163.

Gore C, Custovic A, Tannock G, Munro K, Kerry G, Johnson K, Peterson C, Morris J, Chaloner C, Murray CS, et al. 2012.Treatment and secondary prevention effects of the probiotics *Lactobacillus paracasei* or *Bifidobacterium lactis* on early infant eczema: Randomized controlled trial with follow-up until age 3 years. Clin Exp Allergy. 42:112-122.

Gotcheva V, Hristozova E, Hristozova T, Guo M, Roshkova Z and Angelov A. 2002. Assessment of potential probiotic properties of lactic acid bacteria and yeast strains. Fd Biotechnol. 16: 211-225.

Grahn E. 1994. Interference of a *Lactococcus lactis* strain on the human gut flora and its capacity to pass the stomach and intestine. Scand J Nutr. 38: 2-4.

Gratia A. 1925. Sur unremarquable example d' antagonisme entre deux souches de colibacille CR Seances Soc Biol Fil. 93: 1040-1041.

Greene JD, Klaenhammer TR. 1994. Factors involved in adherence of lactobacilli to human Caco 2 cells. Appl Environ Microbiol. 60:4487-4494.

Gruber C, Wendt M, Sulser C, Lau S, Kulig M, et al. 2007. Randomized placebo-controlled trial of *Lactobacillus rhamnosus* GG as treatment of atopic dermatitis in infancy. Allergy. 62(11):1270-1276.

Guandalini S, Pensabene M and Zikri MA. 2000. *Lactobacillus* GG administered in oral rehydration solution to children with acute diarrhoea: a multicenter European study. J Pediatr Gastroenterol Nutr. 30:54-60.

Guarino A, Berni Canani R, Spagnuolo MI, Albano F, Di Benedetto L.1997. Oral bacterial therapy reduces the duration of symptoms and of viral excretion in children with mild diarrhea. J Pediatr Gastroenterol Nutr.25: 516-519.

Guerin D, Vuillemard JC, Subirade M.2003. Protection of bifidobacteria encapsulated in polysaccharide-protein gel beads against gastric juice and bile. J Fd Protect. 66:2076-2084.

Guerin-Danan C, Chabanet C, Pedone C, et al. 1998. Milk fermented with yogurt cultures and *Lactobacillus casei* compared with yogurt and gelled milk: influence on intestinal microflora in healthy infants. Am J Clin Nutr.67:111-7.

Guessas B and Kihal M. 2004. Characterization of lactic acid bacteria isolated from Algerian arid zone raw goats milk. Afr J Biotechnol. 3: 339-342.

Guilian Y, Jiang Y, Yang W, Du F, Yao Y, Shi C and Wang C. 2015. Effective treatment of hypertension by recombinant *Lactobacillu splantarum* expressing angiotensin converting enzyme inhibitory peptide. Microb Cell Fact.14:202.

Gunasekara R, Casteleyn C, Bossier P and Van den Broeck W. 2012. Comparative stereological study of the digestive tract of *Artemia franciscana* nauplii fed with yeasts differing in cell wall composition. Aquaculture. 324-325: 64-69.

Gupta R, Munoz JC, Garg P, Masri G, Nahman NS Jr, Lambiase LR. 2007. Mediastinal pancreatic pseudocyst–a case report and review of the literature. MedGenMed. 9:8.

Gupta V and Garg R.2009. Probiotics. Ind J Med Microbiol. 27:202-209.

Gupta, S and Abu-Ghannam N. 2012. Probiotic fermentation of plant based products: Possibilities and opportunities. Crit Rev Fd Sci Nutr. 52(2): 183-199.

Guyonnet D, Chassany O and Ducrotte P, et al. 2007. Effect of fermented milk containing *Bifidobacterium animalis* DN-173 010 on the health-related quality of life and symptoms in irritable bowel syndrome in adults in primary care: a multicentre, randomized, double-blind, controlled trial. Aliment Pharmacol Ther.26:475-486.

Ha Y L, Grimm N K and Pariza M W. 1987. Anticarcinogens from fried ground beef: heat-altered derivatives of linoleic acid. Carcinogenesis. 8: 1881-1887.

Halpern G M, Vruwink K G, Van de Water J, Keen C L and Gershwin M E. 1991. Influence of long-term yoghurt consumption in young adults. Int J Immunother. 7:205-210.

Hamer HM, Jonkers D, Venema K, Vanhoutvin S, Troost FJ and Brummer RJ. 2008. The role of butyrate on colonic function. Alim Pharm Thera.27 (2):104-119.

Hamilton-Miller J.M.T. 2003. The role of probiotics in the treatment and prevention of *Helicobacter pylori* infection. Inter J Antimicrob Agents. 360-366.

Hammer HF, Petritsch W, Pristautz H and Krejs GJ.1996. Evaluation of the pathogenesis of flatulence and abdominal cramps in patients with lactose malabsorption. Wien Klin Wochenschr.108: 175-179.

Hammes WP. 2005. Microbial ecology of cereal fermentations. Trends Fd Sci. Technol. 16:4-11.

Hampson DJ.1994. Postweaning *Escherichia coli* diarrhea in pigs.Gyles C L (ed.): *Escherichia coli* in Domestic Animals and Humans. London: CABI. 171-791.

Harms H K, Bertele-Harms R M and Bruer-Kleis D.1987. Enzyme-substitution therapy with the yeast. Saccharomyces cerevisiae in congenital sucrase-isomaltase deficiency. N Engl J Med. 316:1306-1309.

Harty D W, Oakey H J, Patrikakis M, Hume E B and Knox KW.1994. Pathogenic potential of *lactobacilli*. Int JFd Microbiol. 24: 179-189.

Hasler CM. 1998. A new look at an ancient concept.ChemInd.84-89.

Hatakka K, Savilahti E, Ponka A, et al. 2001.Effect of long term consumption of probiotic milk on infections in children attending day care centres: double blind, randomised trial. BMJ 322 (7298):1327.

Havenaar R and Huisin't Veld JHJ. 1992. Probiotics: A general view of Lactic Acid Bacteria. Immunomodulatory effect on immune response in Health and Disease. Ed. BJB Wood. Elsevier App Sc Barking. 1: 151-170.

Hayatsu H, Inoue K, Ohta H, Nama H, Togawa K, Hayatsu T, Makita M and Wataya Y. 1981. Inhibition of the mutagenecity of cooked beef basic fraction by its acidic fraction. Mut Res. 91: 437-442.

Hegde N V, Cook ML, Wolfgang DR, Love BC, Maddox CC and Jayarao BM. 2005. Dissemination of *Salmonellaenterica* sub sp. enterica *Serovar Typhimurium* var. *Copenhagen* clonal types through a contract heifer-raising operation. J Clin Microbiol.43:4208-4211.

Hekmat S and Reid G. 2006. Sensory properties of probiotic yogurt are comparable to standard yogurt. Nutri Res. 26: 163-166.

Hekmat S and Reid G.2007. Survival of *Lactobacillus reuteri* RC-14 and *Lactobacillus rhamnosus* GR-1 in milk. Int J Fd Sci Tech. 42: 615-619.

Hekmat S and Soltani H. 2009. Growth and survival of *Lactobacillus reuteri* RC-14 and *Lactobacillus rhamnosus* GR-1 in yogurt for use as a functional food. Innov Food Sci Emerg Technol.10:293-96.

Hellström AM, Almgren A, Carlsson NG, Svanberg U and Andlid TA. 2012. Degradation of phytate by Pichia kudriavzevii TY13 and *Hanseniaspora guilliermondii* TY14 in Tanzanian togwa. Int J Fd Microbiol. 153: 73-77.

Hellström AM, Vázques-Juárez R, Svanberg U and Andlid TA. 2010. Biodiversity and phytase capacity of yeasts isolated from Tanzanian togwa. Inter J Fd Microbiol. 136: 352-358.

Henneberg W.1904. Zur Kenntnis der Milchsaurebakterien der Brennerei-Maische, derMilch, des Bieres, der Presshefe, der Melasse, des Sauerkohls, der Sauren Gurken und desSauerteigs; sowie einige Bemerkungen uber die Milchsaurebakterien des menssschlishen Magens. Zentbl Bakt. ParasitKde Abt. II;11:15.

Hepner G, Fried R and St Jeor S. 1979. Hypocholesterolemic effect of yogurt and milk. Am J Clin Nutr. 32: 19-24.
Heyman M and MénardS.2002. Probiotic microorganisms: how they affect intestinal pathophysiology. Cell Mol Life Sci. 59: 001-15.
Hill MJ.1983. Bacterial adaptation to lactase deficiency. In: Milk intolerances and rejection. Basel, Switzerland: Karger, Ed. Delmont J. 1983:22-26.
Hilton E, Isenberg HD, Alperstein P, France K and Borenstein MT.1992. Ingestion of yogurt containing *Lactobacillus acidophilus* as prophylaxis for candidal vaginitis. Ann Int Med .116(5): 353-357.
Hirayama K and Rafter J. 2000. The role of probiotic bacteria in cancer prevention. Microbes Infec. 2:681-686.
Hirose Y, Murosaki S, Yamamoto Y, Yoshikai Y, Tsuru T.2006. Daily intake of heat-killed *Lactobacillus plantarum* L-137 augments acquired immunity in healthy adults. J Nutr.136 (12):3069-3073.
Hitti and Miranda. 2006. Probiotics May Help Stressed Gut. WebMD. Retrieved. 10-24.
Hokanson JE and Austin MA.1996. Plasma triglyceride level is a risk factorfor cardiovascular disease independent of high-density lipoprotein cholesterol level: a meta-analysis of population-based prospective studies. J Cardiovasc Risk. 3(2): 213-219.
Holzapfel W H and Schillinger U. 2002. Introduction to pre- and probiotics. Fd Res. Int. 35: 109 -116.
Holzapfel W H, Haberer P, Geisen R, Bjorkroth J and Schillinger U. 2001. Taxonomy and important features of probiotic microorganisms in food and nutrition. Am J Clin Nutr. 73(s): 365s- 373s.
Holzapfel WH, Haberer P, Geisen R, Björkroth J and Schillinger U. 2001. Taxonomy and important features of probiotic microorganisms in food and nutrition1, 2, 3, 4. Am. J Clin Nutr. 73(2): 365s-373s.
Hoppe B, Beck B, Gatter N, von Unruh G, Tischer A, Hesse A, et al. 2006. Oxalobacterformigenes: A potential tool for the treatment of primary hyperoxaluria type1. Kidney Int.70:1305-1311.
Hove H, Nordgaard-Andersen I, Mortensen PB. 1994. Effect of lactic acid bacteria on the intestinal production of lactate and short-chain fatty acids and the absorption of lactose. Am J Clin Nutr.59:74-79.
Howard JC1, Reid G, Gan BS. 2004. Probiotics in surgical wound infections: current status. Clin Invest Med.27 (5):274-281.
Hubalek Z. 2003. Protectants used in the cryopreservation of microorganisms. Cryobiol. 46: 205-229.
Hudault S, Bridonneau C, Raibaud P, Chabanet C and Vial MF. 1994. Relationship between intestinal colonization of *Bifidobacterium bifidum* in infants and the presence of exogenous and endogenous growth-promoting factors in their stools. Pediatr Res. 35(6):696-700.
Human colonic bacteria: role in nutrition, physiology, and pathology. Boca Raton, FL: CRC Press.
Huys R, Llewellyn -Hughes J, Olson P D, et al. 2006. Small subunit rDNA and Bayesian inference reveal Pectenophilusornatus (Copepoda incertae sedis) as highly transformed Mytilicolidae, and support assignment of *Chondracanthidae* and Xarifiidae to *Lichomolgoidea* (Cyclopoida). Biol J Linn Soc.87:403-425.
Ip C, Chin S F, Scimeca J A and Pariza M W.1991. Mammary cancer prevention byconjugated dienoic derivative of linoleic acid. Cancer Res. 51: 6118-6124.
Ishibashi N and Yamazaki S. 2001. Probiotics and safety1, 2, 3. Am J Clin Nutr .2001. 73(2): 465s-470s.

Isolauri E, Majamaa H, Arvola T, Rantala I, Virtanen E and Arvilommi H. 1993. *Lactobacillus casei* strain GC reverses increased intestinal permeability induced by cow milk in suckling rats. Gastroenterol.105: 1643-1650.
Isolauri E, Sütas Y, Kankaanpää P, Arvilommi H, Salminen S.2001. Probiotics: effects on immunity. Am J Clin Nutr. 73(2 Suppl):444S-450S.
Isolauri E. et al. 2008. Probiotics: use in allergic disorders: a Nutrition, Allergy, Mucosal Immunology, and Intestinal Microbiota (NAMI) Research Group Report. J Clin Gastroenter. 42: 91-96.
Ito M, Oshishi K, Yoshida Y, Yokoi W and Sawada H. 2003. Antioxidative effects of lactic acid bacteria on the colonic mucosa of iron-overloaded mice. JAgric Fd Chem. 51: 4456 4460.
Ito M, Sawada H, Ohishi K, Yoshida Y, Yokoi W, Watanabe T and Yokokura T. 2001. Suppressive effects of Bifidobacteria on lipid peroxidation in the colonic mucosa of iron-overloaded mice. J Dairy Sci. 84: 1583-1589.
Jack RW, Tagg JR and Ray B.1995. Bacteriocins of gram positive bacteria. Microbiol Rev. 59:179.
Jacobsen CN, NielsenVR, Hayford AE, Moller PL, Michaelsen KF, Paerregaard A, Sandstrom B, Tvede M and Jacobsen M. 1999. Screening of probiotic activities of forty seven strains of *Lactobacillus* spp. by *in vitro* techniques and evaluation of the colonization ability of five selected strains in humans. Appl Environ Microbiol. 65: 4949-4956.
Jacques N and Casaregola S. 2008. Safety assessment of dairy microorganisms: The hemiascomycetous yeasts. Intern J Fd Microbiol.126: 321-326.
Jakobsen M and Narvhus J. 1996. Yeasts and their possible beneficial and negative effects on the quality of dairy products. Int Dairy J. 6: 755-768.
Jamuna M and Jeevaratnam K.2004. Isolation and partial characterisation of bacteriocins from Pediococcus species. Appl Microbiol Biotechnol. 65(4): 433-439.
Jaspers DA, Massey LW, Luedecke LO.1984. Effect of consuming yogurts prepared with three culture strains on human serum lipoproteins. J Fd Sci. 49: 1178-1181.
Jauhiainen T, Collin M, Narva M, Cheng ZJ, Poussa T, Vapaatalo H, Korpela R. 2005a. Effect of long-term intake of milk peptides and minerals on blood pressure and arterial function in spontaneously hypertensive rats. Milchwissenschaft. 60:358-362.
Jauhiainen T, Vapaatalo H, Poussa T, Kyronpalo S, Rasmussen M, Korpela R. 2005b. *Lactobacillus helveticus* fermented milk lowers blood pressure in hypertensive subjects in 24-h ambulatory blood pressure measurement. Am J Hypertens.18:1600-1605.
Jennifer M and Sinderen D V. 2014. Current taxonomy of phages infecting lactic acid bacteria. Front Microbiol. 5: 7.
Jensen H., Roos S., Jonsson H., Rud I., Grimmer S., Van Pijkeren J. P., et al. (2014). Role of *Lactobacillus reuteri* cell and mucus-binding protein A (CmbA) in adhesion to intestinal epithelial cells and mucus *in vitro*. Microbiology 160 671-681.
Jespersen L.2003. Occurrence and taxonomic characteristics of strains of Saccharomyces cerevisiae predominant in African indigenous fermented foods and beverages. FEMS Yeast Res. 3: 191-200.
Jha P, et al. 1995. The antioxidant vitamins and cardiovascular disease. Annals Inter Med. 123 (11)1: 860-872.
Jhonson T, Nikkila P, Toivonen L, Rosenqvist H and Laakso S. 1995. Cellular fatty acid profile of *Lactobacillus* and *Lactococcus* strains in relation to the oleic acid content of the cultivation medium. App Environ Microbiol. 61: 4497-4499.
Jin LZ, Ho YW, Abdullah N and Jalaludin S.1998. Growth performance, intestinal microbial populations and serum cholesterol of broilers diets containing *Lactobacillus* cultures. Poultry Sci. 77: 1259-1265.
John RP and Nampoothiri MK. 2008. Strain improvement of *Lactobacillus delbruekii* using nitrous acid mutation for L-lactic acid production. World J Microbiol Biotechnol. 24: 3105-3109.

Johnson EA, Nelson JH and Johnson M. 1990. Microbiological safety of cheese made from heat-treated milk. Part I Executive summary, introduction and history. J Fd Protection 53: 441-452.

Johnson et al. 1994. Saccharomyces cerevisiae contains four fatty acid activation (FAA) genes: an assessment of their role in regulating protein N-myristoylation and cellular lipid metabolism. J Cell Biol. 127(3):751-762.

Johnson JD.1981. The regional and ethnic distribution of lactose malabsorption. Adaptive and genetic hypotheses. In: Paige DM, Bayless TM (Eds.) Lactose digestion. Clinical and nutritional implications. Baltimore: Johns Hopkins University Press: 11-22.

Johnson LM et al. 1990. Genetic evidence for an interaction between SIR3 and histone H4 in the repression of the silent mating loci in Saccharomyces cerevisiae. Proc Natl Acad Sci U S A. 87(16):6286-90.

Joneja, Kitts D, Yuan Y, Joneja J, et al. 1997. Adverse reactions to food constituents: allergy, intolerance, and autoimmunity. Can J Physiol Pharmacol.75:241-254.

Jones PJ. 2002. Clinical nutrition: 7. Functional foods – more than just nutrition. CMAJ. 11; 166(12): 1555-1563.

Juránek I and Bezek S. 2005.Controversy of Free Radical Hypothesis: Reactive Oxygen Species - Cause or Consequence of Tissue Injury?Gen. Physiol. Biophys. 24:263–278.

Kabat GC, Chang CJ, Sparano JA, et al. 1997. Urinary estrogen metabolites and breast cancer: a case-control study. Cancer Epidemiol Biomarkers Prev.6 (7):505-509.

Kaila M, Isolauri E, Soppi E,Virtanen E,Laine S and Arvilommi H. 1992. Enhancement of the circulating antibody secreting cell response in human diarrhea by a human *Lactobacillus* strain. Pediatr Res. 32:141-144.

Kailasapathy K and Supraidi D. 1996. Effect of whey protein concentrate on the survival of *L.acidophilus* inlactose hydrolyzed yoghurt during refrigerated storage. Milchwissenschaft. 51: 565-568.

Kailasapathy K, Harmstorf I and Phillips M. 2008. Survival of *Lactobacillus acidophilus* and *Bifidobacterium animalis* ssp lactis in stirred fruit yogurts. LWT-Fd Sci Technol. 41:1317 1322.

Kailasapathy K. 2013. Commercial sources of probiotic strains and their validated and potential health benefits: a review. Intern J Fermn Fds.2 (1):1-17.

Kailasapathy K. and Chin J. 2000. Survival and therapeutic potential of probiotic organisms with reference to *Lactobacillus acidophilus* and *Bifidobacterium* spp. Immunol Cell Biol. 78: 80-88.

Kaizu H, Sasaki M, Nakajima H and Suzuki Y. 1993. Effect of antioxidative lactic acid bacteria on rats fed a diet deficient in vitamin E. J Dairy Sci. 46: 2493-2499.

Kalaiselvan V, Kalaivani M, Vijayakumar A, Sureshkumar K and K.Venkateskumar. 2010. Current knowledge and future direction of research on soy isoflavones as a therapeutic agents. Pharmacogn Rev. 4(8): 111-117.

Kalliomäki M, Salminen S, Arvilommi H, Kero P, Koskinen P and Isolauri E. 2001. Probiotics in primary prevention of atopic disease: a randomised placebo-controlled trial. Lancet. 7; 357 (9262): 1076-1079.

Kalliomäki M, Salminen S, Poussa T, Isolauri E. 2007. Probiotics during the first 7 years of life: A cumulative risk reduction of eczema in a randomized, placebo-controlled trial. J. Allergy Clin Immunol.119:1019-1021.

Kalliomaki MA and Isolauri E. 2004. Probiotics and down regulation of the allergic response. Immunol Allergy Clin. North Am. 24:739-752.

Kampman E, Goldbohm RA, Van Den Brandt PA, Van T, Veer P.1994.Fermented dairy products, calcium and colorectal cancer in the Netherlands cohort study. Cancer Res. 54:3186-3190.

Kankaanpaa P, Young B, Kallio H, Isolauri E and Salminen S. 2004. Effects of polyunsaturated fatty acids in growth medium on lipid composition and on physicochemical surface properties of *Lactobacilli*. Appl Environ Microbiol. 70: 129-136.
Kastner S, Perreten V, Bleulera H, Hugenschmidt G, Lacroix C, Meile L. 2006. Syst Appl Microbiol. 29:145-155.
Kaur I P, Chopra K and Saini A. 2002. Probiotics: Potential pharmaceutical applications. Eur J Pharma Sci.15:1-9.
Kechagia M, Basoulis D, Dimitriadi D, Skarmoutsou N and Fakiri E. 2013. Health benefits of probiotics. 1-7.
Kelly WJ, Davey G P and Ward LJH. 1998. Characterization of Lactococci isolated from minimally processed fresh fruit and vegetables. Int J Fd Microbiol. 45: 85-92.
Khani S, Hosseini M, Hamideh, Mohammad T, MohammadR N, Fooladi A I, Abbas. 2012. Probiotics as an Alternative Strategy for Prevention and Treatment of Human Diseases: A Review.Inflammation & Allergy-Drug Targets (Formerly Current Drug Targets Inflammation & Allergy).11(2):79-89.
Kilara A and Shahani KM. 1975. Lactase activity of cultured and acidified dairy products. J Dairy Sci. 59: 2031-2035.
Kim HS, Gilliland SE.1983. *Lactobacillus acidophilus* as a dietary adjunct for milk to aid lactose digestion in humans. J Dairy Sci. 66:959-966.
Kim J Y, Choi Y O, Ji G E. 2008. Effect of oral probiotics (*Bifidobacterium lactis* AD011 and Lactobacillus acidophilus AD031) administration on ovalbumin-induced food allergy mouse model. J Microbiol Biotechnol. 18:1393-1400.
Kim Ji H, Maeda T and Morita N. 2005. Application of polished-graded wheat grains for Sourdough bread. Cereal Chem. 82:144-151.
Kim YG, Moon JT, Lee KM, Chon NR and Park H. 2006.The effects of probiotics on symptoms of irritable bowel syndrome. Korean J Gastroenterol. 47:413-419.
Kimito H, Nomura M, Kobayash M, Okamoto T and Ohmomo S.2004. Identification and probiotic characteristics of *Lactococcus strain* from plant materials. Jpn Agr Res Q. 38: 111-117.
Kimito H. 2000. *In vitro* studies on probiotic properties of Lactococci. Milchwissenshaft 55: 245-249.
Kimoto H, Ohmomo S and Okamoto T. 2002. Cholesterol removal from media by Lactococci. J Dairy Sci. 85: 3182-3188.
King VAE and Su JT. 1993. Dehydration of *Lactobacillus acidophilus*. Process Biochem. 28: 47-52.
Kirjavainen PV, Salminen S J, Isolauri E. 2003. Probiotic bacteria in the management of atopic disease: underscoring the importance of viability. 223-226.
Kitchell A G and Ingram M.1963. Vacuum packed sliced Wiltshire bacon. Fd Process and Packag. 32: 3.
Klaenhammer TR and Kullen MJ.1999. Selection and design probiotics. Int J Food Microbiol. 50:45-57.
Klaver FAM and Van der Meer R. 1993. The assumed estimation of cholesterol removal by Lactobacilli and *Bifidobacterium bifidum* is due to their bile salt decojugation activity. Applied and environmental microbiology 59:1120-1124.
Kodali VP, Das S and SenR. 2009. An exopolysaccharide from aprobiotic: Biosynthesis dynamic, composition and emulsifying activity. Food Res. Int. 42:695-699.
Kolars JC, Levitt MD, Aouji M, Savaiano DA. 1984. Yogurt–an autodigesting source of lactose. N Engl J Med. 310:1-3.
Korbekandi H, A M Mortazavian and Iravani S. 2011. Technology and stability of probiotic in fermented milks. In Probiotic and Prebiotic Foods: Technology, Stability and Benefits to

the human health pp. 131-169; Shah, N., A.G. Cruz andJ.A.F Faria (Eds.) Nova Science Publishers, New York.

Kos B, Suskovic J, Vukovic S, Simpraga M, Frece J and Matosic S. 2003. Adhesion and aggregation ability of probiotic strain *Lactobacillus acidophilus* M92. J Appl Microbiol. 94: 981-987.

Kosikowski F and MistryVV. 1997. Cheese and fermented milk foods-origins and principles. Wesport, CT, USA: F V Kosikowksi Llc, 1: 87-108.

Kotzamanidis C, Kourelis A, Litopoulou-Tzanetaki E, Tzanetakis N and Yiangou M. 2010. Evaluation of adhesion capacity, cell surface traits and immunomodulatory activity of presumptive probiotic *Lactobacillus strains*. Int J Fd Microbiol. 140: 154-163.

Kotzampassi K, Giamarellos-Bourboulis EJ, Voudouris A, Kazamias P and Eleftheriadis E. 2006. Benefits of a synbiotic formula (Synbiotic 2000Forte) in critically ill trauma patients: early results of a randomized controlled trial. World J Surg. 30:1848-1855.

Kourelis A, Kotzamanidis C, Litopoulou-Tzanetaki E, Scouras Z G, Tzanetakis N and Yiangou M. 2010. Preliminary probiotic selection of dairy and human yeast strains. J. Biol. Res. (Thessalon.) 13: 93-104.

Krasaekoopt W, Bhandari B, Deeth H. 2004. The influence of coating materials on some properties of alginate beads and survivability of microencapsulated probiotic bacteria. Int Dairy J.14:737-743.

Kris-Etherton PN, Krumholz HM, LaRosa J, Ockene IS, Pearson TA, Reed J, Washington R, Smith SC. 1998. Primary prevention of coronary heart disease: guidance from Framingham: a statement for healthcare professionals from the AHA Task Force on Risk Reduction. American Heart Association. Circulation. 12:97(18):1876-1887.

Kruis W, Chrubasik S, Boehm S, Stange C and Schulze J. 2012. A double-blind placebo-controlled trial to study therapeutic effects of probiotic Escherichiacoli Nissle 1917 in subgroups of patients with irritable bowel syndrome. Int J Colorectal Dis. 27(4):467-474.

Kuhn C, Titze A, Lorenz CA.1996. Are viable microorganisms essential for the enhancement of intestinal hydrolysis of lactose by the β-galactosidase of fermented milk products? IDF Nutri Newsletter 5:38.

Kuitunen M. 2013. Current Opinion in Allergy and Clinical Immunology. Probiotics and Prebiotics in Preventing Food Allergy and Eczema Disclosures. Curr Opin Allergy Clin Immunol.13 (3):280-286.

Kuitunen M. et al. 2009. Probiotics prevent IgE-associated allergy until age 5 years in cesarean-delivered children but not in the total cohort. The J Allergy Clin Immunol.123: 335-341.

Kukkonen K, Nieminen T, Poussa T, Savilahti E, Kuitunen M. 2006. Effect of probiotics on vaccine antibody responses in infancy-a randomized placebo-controlled double-blind trial. Pediatr Allergy Immunol. 17(6):416-421.

Kukkonen K. et al. 2008. Long-term safety and impact on infection rates of postnatal probiotic and prebiotic (synbiotic) treatment: randomized, double-blind, placebo-controlled trial. Pediatrics.122: 8-12.

Kulisaar T, Zilmer M, Mikelsaar M, Vihalemm T, Annuk H, Kairane C, Kilk A. 2002.Two antioxidative strains as promising probiotics. Int. J. Fd Microbiol. 72: 215-224.

Kullisaar T, Songisepp E, Mikelsaar M, Zilmer K, Vihalemm T and Zilmer M. 2003. Antioxidative probiotic fermented goats' milk decreases oxidative stress-mediated atherogenicity in human subjects. Br J Nutr. 90: 449-456.

Kumar M, Nagpal R, Kumar R, Hemalatha R, Verma V, Kumar A, Chakraborty C, Singh B, Marotta F, Jain S and Yadav H. 2012. Cholesterol-lowering probiotics as potential biotherapeutics for metabolic diseases. Exp Diabetes Res. 2012:902-917.

Kumura H, Tanoue Y, Tsukahara M, Tanaka T and Shimazaki K.2004. Screening of dairy yeaststrains for probiotic applications. J Dairy Sci. 87:4050-4056.

Kurtzman CP, Fell JW and Boekhout T. 2011. Gene Sequence Analyses and other DNA-Based Methods for Yeast Species Recognition. In: The Yeasts, a Taxonomic Study, Elsevier. B.V: 87-110.

La Ragione RM, Casula G, Cutting SM and Woodward M J. 2001. *Bacillus subtilis* spores competitively exclude Escherichia coli O78:K80 in poultry. Veter Microbiol. 79: 133 142.

Lamothe F and Boullier S. 2002. Interactions between gut microflora and digestive mucosalimmunity, and strategies to improve digestive health in young rabbits. Proceedings - 8th World Rabbit Congress - September 7-10, 2004 - Puebla, Mexico.

Lamsal BP and Faubion JM. 2009. The beneficial use of cereal and cereal components in probiotic foods. Fd Rev Intern. 25(2): 103-114.

Lasser RB, Bond JH and LevittMD.1975. The role of intestinal gas infunctional abdominal pain. New Engl J Med. 293: 524-526.

Lee B and Bak Y. 2011. Irritable bowel syndrome, gut microbiota and probiotics. J Neurogastroenterol Motil. 17: 252-266.

Lee J, Seto D and Bielory L. 2008. Meta-analysis of clinical trials of probiotics for prevention and treatment of pediatric atopic dermatitis. J Allergy Clin Immunol. 121(1):116 -121.

Lee KY and Heo TR. 2000. Survival of *Bifidobacterium longum* immobilized in calcium alginate beads in simulated gastric juices and bile salt solution. Appl Environ Microbiol. 66: 869-873.

Lee YK and Salminen S. 1995. The coming of age of probiotics. Trends Fd Sci. Technol. 6: 241-245.

Lee YK, Nomoto K, Salminen S and Gorbach SL.1999. Handbook of Probiotics," John Wiley & Sons, Inc. N.Y.

Lee YK, Puong KY, Ouwehand AC and Salminen S. 2003.Displacement of bacterial pathogens from mucus and Caco-2 cell surface by lactobacilli. J Med Microbiol. 52: 925-930.

Leite AMO, Miguel MA, Peixoto RS, Rosado AS, Silva JT and Paschoalin V M. 2013. Microbiological, technological and therapeutic properties of kefir: a natural probiotic beverage. Braz J Microbiol. 44(2): 341-349

Leopold and Eileler D.2000. Basic coating polymer for the colon-specific drug discovery in inflammatory bowel disease. Drug Dev Ind Pharm. 26:1239-1246.

Leporanta K. 2001. Developing fermented milks into functional foods. InnovFd Technol. 46-47.

Lerebours E, N'Djitoyap Ndam C, Lavoine A, Hellot MF, Antoine JM and Colin R.1989. Yogurt and fermented-then-pasteurized milk: effects of short-term and long-term ingestion on lactose absorption and mucosal lactase activity in lactase-deficient subjects. Am J Clin Nutr. 49:823-827.

Leroy F, Falony G and Vuyst L.2008. Latest Developments in Probiotics. In: Toldra F, Ed. Meat Biotechnology. Brussels, Belgium: Springer. 217-229.

Lesbros-Pantoflickova D, Corthe'sy-Theulaz I and Blum AL.2007. Helicobacterpylori and probiotics. J Nutr. 137(Suppl2) 812S-8128S.

Levine GN, Keaney JF, Vita JA. 1995. Cholesterolreduction in cardiovascular dis280 ease. Clinical benefitsand possible mechanisms. New England J Med. 332: 512-521.

Levitt MD, Gibson GR, Christl SU.1995. Gas metabolism in the large intestine. In: Gibson GR, MacFarlane GT (Eds.)

Lewanika SJ, Abratt VR, Macfarlane GT and Macfarlane S.2007. *Lactobacillus gasseri* Gasser AM63T degrades oxalate in a multistage continuous culture stimulatorof the human colonic microbiota. FEMS Microbiol Ecol. 61(1):110-120.

Lewanika T R, Reid S J, AbrattV R, Macfarlane G T and Macfarlane S. 2007. *Lactobacillus gasseri* Gasser AM63T degrades oxalate in a multistage continuous culture simulator of the human colonic microbiota. FEMS Microbiol Ecol. 61(1): 110-120.

Lian WC, Hsiao HC and Chou CC. 2003. Viability of microencapsulated *Bifidobacteria* in simulated gastric juice and bile solution. Int J Fd Microbiol. 86: 293-301.

Liliana S C and Aida Rodriguez de S. 2006. Lactic acid production by a strain of *Lactococcus lactis* subs lactis isolated from sugar cane plants. J Biotechnol. 9: 40-45.

Lin M, Savaiano D and Harlender S. 1991. Influence of non-fermented dairy products containing bacterial starter cultures on lactose maldigestion in humans. J Dairy Sci. 74: 87 95.

Lin MY and Chang FY. 2000. Antioxidative effect of intestinal bacteria *Bifidobacterium longum* ATCC15708 and *Lactobacillus acidophilus* ATCC 4356. Dig Dis Sci 45: 1617-1622.

Lin MY and Yen CL. 1999. Antioxidative ability of lactic acid bacteria. J Agric Fd Chem. 47: 1460-1466.

Lin MY, Savaiano D, Harlander S.1991. Influence of nonfermented dairy products containing bacterial starter cultures on lactose maldigestion in humans. J Dairy Sci. 74:87-95.

Lin MY. 1995. *In vivo* lactose digestion by *Lactobacillus acidophilus*. J Chin Nutr Soc. 20:147-156.

Lin S Y, Ayres J W, Winkler W and Sandine WE.1989. *Lactobacillus* effects on cholesterol: in vitro and in vivo results. J Dairy Res. 72: 2885-2889.

Link-Amster H, Rochat F, Saudan K Y, Mignot O and Aeschlimann J M. 1994. Modulation of a specific humoral immune response and changes in intestinal flora mediated through fermented milk intake. FEMS Immunol Med Microbiol. 10: 55-63.

Liong MT.2007. Probiotics: A critical Review of Their Potential Role as Antihypertensives, Immune Modulators,

Lislie SB, Israeli E, Lighthart B, Crowe JH and Crowe LM. 1995. Trehalose and sucrose protect both membranes and

Liu W, Wang Y, Yu Z and Bao J.2012. Simultaneous saccharification and microbial lipid fermentation of corn stover by oleaginous yeast *Trichosporon cutaneum*. Bioresour Technol.118:13-18.

Liu Y, Fatheree N, Mangalat N and Rhoads J. 2010. Human-derived probiotic *Lactobacillus reuteri* strains differentially reduce intestinal inflammation. Am J Physiol Gastrointest Liver Physiol. 299: G1087-G1096.

Ljungh A and Wadstrom T (editors). 2009. *Lactobacillus* Molecular Biology: From Genomics to Probiotics. Caister

Logan AC, Venket Rao A, Irani D. 2003.Chronic fatigue syndrome: lactic acid bacteria may be of therapeutic value. Med Hypotheses. 60:915-923.

Lollo P C B, Cruz G, Morato P N, Moura C S, Carvalho-Silva L B, Oliveira C F et al. 2012. Probiotic cheese attenuates exercise-induced immune suppression in Wistar rats. J. Dairy Sci. 95: 3549-3558.

Lonning P E, Johannessen DC, Lien EA, Ekse D, Fotsis T and Adlercreutz H. 1995. Influence of tamoxifen on sex hormones, gonadotrophins and sex hormone binding globulin in postmenopausal breast cancer patients. J Steroid Biochem Mol Biol. 52: 491-496.

Lopandic K, Zelger S, Banszky L K, EliskasesL F and Prillingera H. 2006. Identification of yeasts associated with milk products using traditional and molecular techniques. Fd Microbiol. 23:341-350.

Lopez HW, Ouvry A, Bervas E, Guy G, Messager A, Demigne C and Remsey C. 2000. Strains of lactic acid bacteria isolated from sour doughs degrade phytic acid and improve calcium and magnesium solubility from whole wheat flour. J Agric Fd Chem. 48: 2281 2285.

Lopez RV, Cook RL, Sobel JD. 1990. Emerging role of *Lactobacilli* in the control and maintenance of the vaginal bacterial microflora. Rev Infect Dis. 12:856-872.

López-KleineL, Trubuil A and Monnet V. 2011. Sensitivity Analysis of Protein Role Prediction Methods: Which are the Relevant Data? The Open Genomics J.4: 1-9.

Lorea B M, Kirjavainen P V, Hekmat S and Reid G. 2001. Anti inflammatory effects of probiotic yogurt in inflammatory bowel disease patients. Am J Clin Nutr. 73(2 Suppl) 361 s-364s.

Lourens-Hattingh A and Viljoen BC. 2001. Yogurt as probiotic carrier food. Int Dairy J. 11: 1-17.

Lue KH, Sun HL, Lu KH, Ku MS, Sheu JN, Chan CH and Wang YH. 2012. A trial of adding *Lactobacillus johnsonii* EM1 to levocetirizine for treatment of perennial allergic rhinitis in children aged 7-12 years. Int J Pediatr Otorhinolaryngol. 76(7):994-1001.

Luo P, Hu C, Xie Z, Zhang L, Ren C, Xu Y.2006. PCR-DGGE analysis of bacterial community composition in brackish water *Litopenaeus vannamei* culture system. J Trop Oceanogr. 25:49-53.

Lutgendorff F, Nijmeijer RM, Sandström P A, Trulsson LM, Magnusson KE, Timmerman H M, L. van Minnen P, Rijkers G T, Gooszen HG, Akkermans L MA, Söderholm JD. 2009. Probiotics Prevent Intestinal Barrier Dysfunction in Acute Pancreatitis in Rats via Induction of Ileal Mucosal Glutathione Biosynthesis. Plusone. 4 (2): e4512; 1-13.

Mack DR, Michail S and Wet S. 1999. Probiotics inhibit enteropathogenic *E. coli* adherence in vitro by inducing intestinal mucin gene expression. Am J Physiol. 276: G941-G 950.

Madden JAJ, et al. 2005. Effect of probiotics on preventing disruption of the intestinal microflora following antibiotic therapy: A double blind, placebo controlled pilot study. Int Immunopharmacol. 5(6):1091-1097.

Mahony J, van Sinderen D.2015.Novel strategies to prevent or exploit phages in fermentations, insights from phage-host interactions. Curr Opin Biotechnol.32:8-13.

Majamaa H and Isolauri E. 1997. Probiotics: a novel approach in the management of food allergy. J Allergy Cim Immunol. 99: 179-185.

Majchrzak D, Hartjes B, Hartjes B and Dürrschmid K.2010. Conventional and Probiotic yoghurts differ in the sensory properties, but not in consumer preferences. Journal of Sensory Studies. 25(3):431 - 446.

Makri A, Fakas S, Aggelis G. 2010. Metabolic activities of biotechnological interest in *Yarrowia lipolytica* grown on glycerol in repeated batch cultures. Bioresour Technol. 101: 2351-2358.

Malin M, Verronen P and Korhonen H. 1997. Dietary therapy with *Lactobacillus* GG, bovine colostrums or bovine immune colostrums in patients with juvenile chronic arthritis: mallett evaluation of effect of gut defense mechanisms. Inflammopharmacol. 5: 219-236.

Mallett AK, Bearne CA and Rowland IR. 1989. The influence of incubation pH on the activity of rat and human gut flora enzymes. J Appl Bacteriol. 66: 433-437.

Mann G V and A. Spoerry. 1974. Studies of a surfactant and cholesteremia in the Maasai. Am J Clin Nutr. 27: 464-469.

Manson JE, Colditz GA, Stampfer MJ, Willett WC, Kroleswki AS, Rosner B, Arky RA, Speizer FE, Hennekens CH. 1991. A prospective study of maturity-onset diabetes mellitus and risk of coronary heart disease and stroke in women. Arch Intern Med. 151:1141-1147.

Manson JE, Rimm EB, Colditz GA, Willett WC, Nathan DM, Arky RA, Rosner B, Hennekens CH, Speizer FE, Stampfer MJ.1992. A prospective study of postmenopausal estrogen therapy and subsequent incidence of noninsulin-dependent diabetes mellitus. Ann Epidemiol. 2:665-673.

MAPA: Brasil, Ministério da Agricultura, Pecuária e Abastecimento 2007. Instrução Normativa n° 46 de 23 de outubro de. Regulamento Técnico de Identidade e Qualidade de Leites Fermentados. Diário Oficial da União, Brasília, seção 1, p.5, 24 de outubro de.

Marelli G, Papaleo E and Ferrari A. 2004. *Lactobacilli* for prevention of urogenital infections: a review. Eur Rev Med Pharmacol Sci. 8(2):87-95.

Maria Filomena de Jesus Raposo, Rui Manuel Santos Costa de Morais, and Alcina Maria Miranda Bernardo de Morais. 2013. Bioactivity and Applications of Sulphated Polysaccharides from Marine Microalgae. Mar Drugs. 11(1): 233-252.

Marklinder IM and Lonner C.1992. Fermentation properties of intestinal strains of *Lactobacillus* of a sourdough and yoghurt starter culture in an oat-based nutrition solution. Fd Microbiol. 9: 197-203.

Marschan E, Kuitunen M, Kukkonen K, Poussa T, Sarnesto A, et al. 2008. Probiotics in infancy induce protective immune profiles that are characteristicfor chronic low-grade inflammation. Clin Exp Allergy.38 (4):611- 618.

Marshall RW, Cochran M and Hodgkinson A.1972. Relationships between calcium and oxalic acid intake in the diet and their excretion in the urine of normal and renal-stone forming subjects. Clin. Sci. 43: 91-99.

Marteau P, Cuillerier E, Meance S, Gerhardt MF, Myara A, Bouvier M, Bouley C, Tondu F, Bommelaer G, Grimaud JC. 2002. *Bifidobacterium* animalis strain DN-173 010 shortens the colonic transit time in healthy women: a double-blind, randomized, controlled study. Aliment Pharmacol Ther.16:587-93.

Marteau P, Flourie B, Pochart P, Chastang C, Desjeux JF, Rambaud JC.1990. Effect of the microbial lactase (EC 3.2.1.23) activity in yoghurt on the intestinal absorption of lactose: an in vivo study on lactase-deficient humans. Br J Nutr.64:719.

Marteau P, Minekus M, Havenaar R and Huis In'tVeld JHJ. 1997. Survival of lactic acid bacteria in a dynamic model of the stomach and small intestine: Validation and the effects of bile. J Dairy Sci. 80:1031-1037.

Marteau P, Pochart P, Bouhnik Y and Ramband JC. 1993. The fate and effects of transiting nonpathogenic microrganisms in the human intestine. World Rev Nutr. Diet.74: 1-21.

Marteau P. 2001.Safety aspects of probiotic products. Scandinavian J Nutr. /Naringsforskning. 45:22-24.

Marteau PR, de Vrese M, Cellier CJ and Schrezenmeir J.2001. Protection from gastrointestinal diseases with the use of Probiotics. Am J Clin Nutr. (Suppl.).73:430-436.

Martini M C, Kukielka D and Savalano DA. 1991a. Lactose digestion from yogurt: influence of a meal and additional lactose. Am J Clin Nutr. 53: 1253-1258.

Martini MC, Bolweg G L, Levitt MD and Savaiano DA.1987. Lactose digestion by yoghurt h-galactosidase. Influence of pH and microbial cell integrity. Am J Clin Nutr.45: 432-437.

Martini MC, Lerebours EC, Lin WJ, et al. 1991b. Strains and species of lactic acid bacteria in fermented milks (yogurts): effect on in vivo lactose digestion. Am J Clin Nutr. 54:1041-1046.

Martini MC, Smith DE, Savaiano DA. 1987. Lactose digestion from flavored and frozen yogurts, ice milk and ice cream by lactase-deficient persons. Am J Clin Nutr. 1987. 46:636-640.

Martley F G and Crow V L.1993. Interaction between nonstarter microorganisms during cheese manufacture and ripening. Int Dairy J.3:461-483.

Marttinen A, Haukioja A, Karjalainen S, Nylund L, Satokari R, Öhman C. et al. 2011. Short-term consumption of probiotic lactobacilli has no effect on acid production of supragingival plaque. Clin Oral Investig.16:797-803.

Massey LK, Roman-Smith H and Sutton RAL.1993. Effect of dietary oxalate and calcium on urinary oxalate and risk of formation of calcium oxalate kidney stones. J Am Diet Assoc. 93: 901-906.

Mastromarino P, Vitali B, Mosca L.2013. Bacterial vaginosis: a review on clinical trialswith probiotics.New Microbiologica.36: 229-238.

Matsuzaki T and Chin J.2000. Modulating immune responses with probiotic bacteria. Immunol Cell Biol. 78: 67-73.

Mattila-Sandholm Tand Kauppila T. 1998. Functional Food Research in Europe 3rd Workshop, Fair CT96- 1028, Probdemo, VTT Symposium 187. Haikko, Finland, 125.

Matto J, Fonden R, Tolvanen T, Vonwright A, Vilpponensalmela T, Satokari R, et al. 2006. Intestinal survival and persistence of probiotic *Lactobacillus* and *Bifidobacterium* strains administered in triple-strain yoghurt. Int. Dairy J. 16, 1174-1180.

McBean LD, Miller GD. 1998. Allaying fears and fallacies about lactose intolerance. J Am Diet Assoc.98:671-676.
McDonald P, Edwards RA, Greenhalgh JFD and Morgan CA.2002. Animal Nutrition sixth Ed. Pearson Education Limited (Prentice Hall) U.K. 693. ISBN 0-582-41906-9.
McFarland L, Surawicz C and Greenberg R. 1994. A randomised placebo-controlled trial of *Saccharomyces boulardii* in combination with standard antibiotics for *Clostridium difficile* disease. J Am Med Assoc. 271: 1913-1918.
McFarland LV, Surawicz C M, Greenberg R N, Elmer G W, Moyer K A, Melcher S A, Bowen K E and Cox J L.1995. Prevention of beta-lactam-associated diarrhea by *Saccharomyces* in combination with standard antibiotics for *Clostridium difficile* disease. J. Am. Med Assoc. 271: 1913-1918.
McFarland LV. 2000. Beneficial microbes: health or hazard? Eur J Gastroenterol Hepatol. 12: 1069-1071.
McFarland LV.2006. Meta-analysis of probiotics for the prevention of antibiotic associated diarrhea and the treatment of *Clostridium difficile* disease. Am J Gastroenterol. 101: 812-822.
McFarland LV.2007. Meta-analysis of probiotics for the prevention of traveler's diarrhea.Trav Med InfectDis.5 (2): 97-105.
McGann LE.1978. Differing actions of penetrating and non-penetrating cryoprotective agents. Cryobiol. 15 (4): 382-390.
Medical Hypotheses. 60(6):915-923.
Meneghin F, Fabiano V, Mameli C and Zuccotti GV. 2012. Atopic Dermatitis in Children. Pharmaceuticals (Basel). 5(7): 727-744.
Meneghin F, Fabiano V, Mameli C, Vincenzo Z G, Famularo G, Perluigi M, Pieluigi M, Coccia R, Mastroiacovo P and De Simone C. 2001. Probiotics and Microecology, bacterial vaginosis and probiotics: perspectives for bacteriotherapy. 421-430.
Mensink RP, Aro A, Den Hond E, German JB, Griffin BA, ten Meer HU, Mutanen M, Pannemans D and Stahl W. 2003. Passclaim - Diet-related cardiovascular disease. Eur J Nutr. 42: 16-27.
Messaoudi M, Lalonde R, ViolleN, Javelot H, Desor D,Nejdi A,FrancJÿois Bisson, Rougeot C, Pichelin M, Cazaubiel M and Cazaubiel JM.2011. Assessment of psychotropic-like properties of a probiotic formulation (*Lactobacillus helveticus* R0052 and Bifidobacterium longum R0175) in rats and human subjects. Brit J Nutr. 105:755-764.
Metchnikoff E.1908. The prolongation of life. G.P Putnam's Sons.161.
Meurman JH, Antila H and Salminen S. 1994. Recoveryof lactobacillus strain GG (ATCC 53103) from saliva of healthy volunteers after consumption of yoghurt prepared with the bacterium. Microb Ecol Health Dis. 7:295-298.
Mezaini A, Chihib NE, Bouras AD, Arroume NN and Horne JP. 2009. Antibacterial Activity of Some Lactic Acid Bacteria Isolated from an Algerian Dairy Product. J Environ Public Health. 678495.
Miao S, Mills S, Stanton C, Fitzgerald GF, Roos Y and Roos PR. 2008. Effect of disaccharides on survival during storage of freeze dried probiotics. Dairy Sci Technol. 88: 19-30.
Michail S. 2009.The role of Probiotics in allergic diseases. Allergy Asthma Clin Immunol. 5(1):5.
Michalkiewicz J, Krotkiewski M, Gackowska L, Wyszomirska-Golda M, Helmin-Basa A, Dzierzanowska D and Madalinski K. 2003. Immunomodulatory effects of lactic acid bacteria on human peripheral blood mononuclear cells. Microb Ecol Health Dis. 15:185- 192.
Miller RA and Britigan BE.1997. Role of oxidants inmicrobial physiology. Clin Microbiol Rev. 10: 1-18.
Mills S C, Stanton G, Fitzgerald RP and Ross.2011. Enhancing the stress responses of probiotics for a lifestyle from gut to product and back again.Microbial Cell Fac. S19.

Mishra K, Ojha H and Chaudhury NK. 2012. Estimation of antiradical properties of antioxidants using DPPH assay: A critical review and results. Fd Chemi. 130: 1036-1043.

Mishra S K, Mishra P and Saxena M.2012. Probiotics: An Approach for Better Treatment. Res J Pharma Biol Chem Sci. 3: 1042.

Mohan J C.1990. Preliminary observations on effect of *L. sporogenes* on serum lipid levels in hypercholesterolemic patients. Ind J Med Res. 92: 431-432.

Mombelli B and Gismondo MR. 2000. The use of probiotics in medical practice. Intern J Antimicrob Agents.16:531-536.

Montanarai G, Zambonelli C, Grazia L, Benevelli M and Chiavari C. 2000. Release of beta galactosidase from *Lactobacilli*. Fd Technol Biotech. 38: 129-133.

Monteagudo M A, Aparicioa L R, Rúaa J, Blancoa H M, Navasaa N, ArmestobMRG and Ferrero MA. 2012. *In vitro* evaluation of physiological probiotic properties of different lactic acid bacteria strains of dairy and human origin. J Functional Fds. 4(2):531-541.

Moreira N, Pina C, Mendes F, Couto J A, Hogg T and Vasconcelos I. 2011. Volatile compounds contribution of *Hanseniaspora guilliermondii* and *Hanseniaspora uvarum* during red wine vinifications. Fd Contr. 22:662-667.

Moroti C, Souza Magri LF, de Rezende Costa M, Cavallini DC, Sivieri K. 2012. Effect of the consumption of a new symbiotic shake on glycemia and cholesterol levels in elderly people with type 2 diabetes mellitus. Lipids Health Dis. 11:29.

Muñoz M, Mosquera A, Alméciga-Díaz C J, Melendez A P, Sánchez O F. 2012. Fructooligosaccharides metabolism and effect on bacteriocin production in *Lactobacillus* strains isolated from ensiled corn and molasses. Anaerobe. 18: 321-330.

Nahaisi L, Hatakka K and Savilabtis R. 1986. Effect of long term consumption of a probiotic bacterium *Lactobacillus rhamnosus* in milk on dental carries and carries risk in children. Res. 35(6):412-420.

Naidu AS, Bidlack WR, Clemens RA. 1999. Probiotic spectra of lactic acid bacteria (LAB).Crit Rev Fd Sci Nutr.39 (1):13-126.

NakatsujiT, Kao M C, Fang JY, Zouboulis C C, Zhang L, Gallo R L and Huang C M. 2009. Antimicrobial property of lauric acid against Propionibacterium acnes: Its therapeutic potential for inflammatory acne vulgaris. J Investigative Dermatol. 129: 2480-2488.

Nase L, Hatakka K, Savilahti E, et al. 2001. Effect of long-term consumption of a probiotic bacterium, *Lactobacillus rhamnosus* GG, in milk on dental caries and caries risk in children. Caries Res. 35 (6): 412-420.

Nayak SK and Mukherjee SC. 2011.Screening of gastrointestinal bacteria of Indian major carps for a candidate probiotic species for aquaculture practices. Aquaculture Res. 42(7):1034-1041.

Nemcová R. 1997.Criteria for selection of lactobacilli for probiotic use. Vet Med (Praha). 42(1):19-27.

Newcomer AD, McGill DB, Thomas PJ, Hofmann AF.1978.Tolerance to lactose among lactase deficient American Indians. Gastroenterol.74:44-46.

Ng (2008). Colonization of intestinal microflora: 412-420.

Ng SC, Hart AL, Kamm MA, Stagg AJ and Knight SC.2009. Mechanism of action of probiotics: Recent Adv.15:300-308.

Nguyen T, Nguyen M, Geiger B, Mathiesen G, Eijsink VGH, Peterbauer CK, Haltrich D and Nguyen TH.2015. Heterologous expression of a recombinant lactobacillal beta-galactosidase in *Lactobacillus plantarum*: effect of different parameters on the sakacin P-based expression system.Microb Cell Fact.14: 30.

Nikolic M, López P, Strahinic I, Suárez A, Kojic M, Fernández-García M, et al. 2012. Characterisation of the exopolysaccharide (EPS)-producing *Lactobacillus paraplantarum* BGCG11 and its non-EPS producing derivative strains as potential probiotics. Int. J. Fd Microbiol. 158:155-162.

References 153

Ning X, Cui Y, Yin YN, Zhao X, Yang JW, Wang ZG, Fu N, Tang Y, Wang XH, Liu XW, Wang CL and LuFG. 2011. Effects of two *Lactobacillus* strains on lipid metabolism and intestinal microflora in rats fed a high-cholesterol diet. BMC Complement Altern Med. 11: 53.

Noh DO, Kim SH and Gilliland S E. 1997. Incorporation of cholesterol into the cellular membrane of *Lactobacillus acidophilus* ATCC 43121. J Dairy Sci. 80: 3107-3113.

Novak TE, Lakshmanan Y, Trock BJ, Gearhart JP and Matlaga BR. 2009. Sex prevalence of pediatric kidney stone disease in the United States: an epidemiologic investigation. Urology.74:104-1047.

Noverr MC and Huffnagle GB.2004. Does the microbiota regulate immune responses outside the gut? Trends Microbiol.12 (12):562-568.

O'Grady and G R Gibson. 2007. Chapter 1, Microbiota of the Human Gut (pages 1-15), B. Probiotic Dairy Products. Ed(s): Adnan Tamime Published Online: 16 NOV Print ISBN: 9781405121248 Online ISBN: 9780470995785.

O'Hara AM and Shanahan F. 2007. Mechanisms of action of probiotics in intestinal diseases. Sci World J. 10:7:31-46.

Oberhelman RA, Gilman EH, Sheen P, Taylor DN, Black RE, Cabrera L, Lescano AG, Meza R and Madico G.1999. A placebo-controlled trial of *Lactobacillus* GG to prevent diarrhea in undernourished Peruvian children. J Pediat.134:15-20.

Oberman H and Libudzisz Z. 1998. Fermented Milks. In: Microbiology of Fermented Foods. Wood B.J.B. (Ed.). Blackie Academic and Professional, London. ISBN: 0751402168: 308 350.

Odunfa SA and Oyewole OB.1998.African fermented food. In: Microbiology of Fermented Foods.2.Woods BJ. (Eds.). Elsevier Applied Science Publishers London.

Ogunremi OR, Sanni A and Agrawal R. 2015. Probiotic potentials of yeasts isolated from some cereal-based Nigerian traditional fermented food products. J Appl Microbiol.119(3):797-808.

Oksanen PJ, Salminen S and Saxelin M. 1990. Prevention of travellers' diarrhea by Lactobacillus GG. Annals of Med. 22 (1): 53-56.

Olasupo NA. 2006. Fermentation biotechnology in Africa. In: Fd Biotechnol. 2nd Edition. Shetty K, Paliyath G, Pometto A and Levin RE. (Eds.) CRC Press, Boca Raton.

Olsen GJ, Woese CR, Overbeck R.1994. The winds of (evolutionary) change: breathing new life into microbiology. J Bacteriol.176:1-6.

Omemu AM, Oyewole OB, Bankole MO. 2007.Significance of yeast in the fermentation of maize for Ogi production. Fd Microbiol. 24:571-576.

Ong L and Shah NP. 2008. Influence of probiotic *Lactobacillus acidophilus* and *L. helveticus* on proteolysis, organic acid profiles, and ACE-inhibitory activity of cheddar cheeses ripened at 4, 8, and 12 degrees C. J Fd Sci.73:M111-M120.

Onwulata CI, Rao DR, Vankineni P.1989. Relative efficiency of yogurt, sweet acidophilus milk, hydolyzed-lactose milk, and a commercial lactase tablet in alleviating lactose maldigestion. Am J Clin Nutr.49:1233-1237.

Opinion of the Scientific Steering Committee of the Norwegian Scientific Committee for Food Safety. Combined toxic effects of multiple chemical exposures. Report 1: 2008.available at http://www.vkm.no/eway/library/open Form. aspx?param1=17786¶m5=read).] {178818}

Otieno DO, NP Shah. 2007. Endogenous â-glucosidase and β-galactosidase activities from selected probiotic microorganisms and their role in isoflavone biotransformation in soymilk.103 (4):910-917.

Ouwehand A C, Salminen S and Isolauri E. 2002. Probiotics: an overview of beneficial effects. Antonie Van Leeuwenhoek. 279-289.

Ouwehand A C. 2007. Antiallergic Effects of Probiotics. J. Nutr. 137: 794S-797S.
Ouwehand AC and Salminen SJ. 1998. The health effects of cultured milk products with viable and non-viable bacteria. Int Dairy J. 8:749-758.
Ouwehand AC, Kirjavainen PV, Gronlund MM, Isolauri E and Salminen SJ. 1999a. Adhesion of probiotic micro-organisms to intestinal mucus. Int Dairy J. 9: 623-30.
Ouwehand AC. Kirjavainen PV, Shortt C and Salminen S.1999b. Probiotics: mechanics and established effects. Int Dairy J. 9: 43-52.
Ozdemir O. 2010.Various affects of different probiotic strains in allergic disorders: an update from laboratory and clinical data.Clin Exp Immunol. 160: 295-304.
Pan CL, Zhao YX, Liao SFF, Chen F, QinSY, Wu XS, Zhou H and Huang KH.2011.Effect of Selenium-Enriched Probiotics on Laying Performance, Egg Quality, Egg Selenium Content, and Egg Glutathione Peroxidase Activity. J Agri Fd Chem. 59(21): 11424-11431.
Panoff, J.M., Thammavongs, B., Guéguen, M. 2000. Cryoprotectants lead to Phenotypic Adaptation to Freeze-Thaw Stress in *Lactobacillus delbrueckii* ssp. *bulgaricus* CIP101027T. Cryobiol. 40:264-269.
Pant AR, Graham SM and Allen SJ. 1996. *Lactobacillus* GG and acute diarrhoea in young children in the tropics. J Trop Pediatr. 42:162-165.
Paola M, Vitali B and Luciana. 2013. Bacterial vaginosis: a review on clinical trials with probiotics. New Microbiologica. 36: 229-238.
Pariza M W and Hargraves W A. 1985. A beef-derivatived mutagenesis modulator inhibits initiation of mouse epidermal tumors by 7, 12-dimethylbenz[a] anthracene. Carcinogenesis. 6: 591-593.
Pariza MW, Park Y and Cook ME.2001.The biologically active isomers of conjugated linoleic acid. Prog Lipid Res. 40:283-298.
Park DY, Ahn YT, Park SH, et al. 2013. Supplementation of *Lactobacillus curvatus* HY7601 and *Lactobacillus plantarum* KY1032 in diet-induced obese mice is associated with gut microbial changes and reduction in obesity.PLoS One.8(3):e59470.
Parker RB.1974. Probiotics, the other half of theantibiotics story. Animal Nutri Health. 29:4 8.
Parkouda C, Diawara B, Lowor S, Diako C, Saalia FK, Annan N T, et al. 2011. Volatile compounds of maari, a fermented product from baobab (*Adansoniadigitata* L.) seeds. Afr J Biotechnol. 10:4197-4206.
Parvez S, Lee HC, Kim DS and Kim HY. 2006 a. Bile salt hydrolase and cholesterol removal effect by *Bifidobacterium bifidum* NRRL 1976. World J Microbiol Biotechnol. 22: 455 459.
Parvez S, Malik KA, Kang S A and Kim H Y. 2006 b. Probiotics and their fermented food products are beneficial for health. J Appl Microbiol.100: 1171-1185.
Parvez S, Malik KA, Kang S, Kim H Y. 2005. Probiotics and their fermented food products are beneficial for health. J Appl Microbiol.100:1171-1185.
Passeron T, Lacour J, Fontas E and Ortonne JP.2006. Prebiotics and synbiotics: Two promising approaches for the treatment of atopic dermatitis in children above 2 years. Allergy. 60:431-437.
Patist A and Zoerb H. 2005. Preservation mechanisms of trehalose in food and biosystems. Colloids Surf B. 40: 107-113.
Paton AW, Morona R and Paton JC. 2006. Designer probiotics for prevention of enteric infections. Nature Rev Microbiol. 4: 193-200.
Pedersen A N, Kondrup J and Børsheim E.2013. Health effects of protein intake in healthy adults: a systematic literature review.FdNutr Res.57: 10.3402/fnr.v57i0.21245.
Peera H and Versalovic J. 2013. Effects of probiotics on gut microbiota: mechanisms of intestinal immunomodulation and neuromodulation.TherapAdv Gastroenterol. 6(1): 39-51.

Pelletier C, Bouley C C, Bouttier S, Bourlioux P, Bellon-fontaine MN.1997.Cell surface characteristics of *Lactobacillus casei* sub sp. casei, *Lactobacillus paracasei* sub sp. *paracasei*, and *Lactobacillus rhamnosus* strains. Appl Environ Microbiol. 63(5): 1725-1731.

Peng GC and Hsu CH. 2005.The efficacy and safety of heat-killed Lactobacillusparacasei for treatment of perennial allergic rhinitis induced by house-dust mite. Pediat Allergy Immuno.16 (5): 433-438.

Perapoch J, Planes AM, Querol A, Lopez V, Martinez-Bendayan I, Tormo R, et al. 2000. Fungemia with *Saccharomyces cerevisiae* in two newborns, only one of whom had been treated with ultra-levura. Eur J Clin Microbiol Infect Dis. 19: 468-470.

Perdigon G, de Macias M E, Alvarez S, Oliver G and de Ruiz Holgado AA. 1986. Effect of perorally administered lactobacilli on macrophage activation in mice. Infect Immun.53: 404-410.

Perdigón G, Medici M, Bibas Bonet de Jorat ME, Valverde De,Budeguer M, and Pesce de.1993. Immuno modulating effects of lactic acid bacteria on mucosal and tumoral immunity. Int J Immunother. 9: 29 -52.

Perman JA, Modler S, Olson AC. 1981. Role of pH in production of hydrogen from carbohydrates by colonic bacterial flora. Studies *in vivo* and *in vitro*. J Clin Invest.67: 643- 50.

Perricone M, Bevilacqua AA, Corbo MR and Sinigaglia M. 2014. Technological Characterization and Probiotic traits of Yeasts Isolated from Altamura Sourdough to Select Promising Microorganisms as Functional Starter Cultures for Cereal-Based Products. Fd Microbiol. 38: 26-35.

Perrin Y, Nutten S, Audran R, et al. 2014. Comparison of two oral probiotic preparations in a randomized crossover trial highlights a potentially beneficial effect of *Lactobacillus paracasei* NCC2461 in patients with allergic rhinitis. Clin Transl Allergy. 4(1):1.

Petersson L G, Magnusson K, Hakestam U, Baigi A and Twetman S. 2011. Reversal of primary root caries lesions after daily intake of milk supplemented with fluoride and probiotic lactobacilli in older adults. Acta Odontol Scand. 69: 321-327.

Petti S, Tarsitani G and D'Arca AS. 2001. A randomized clinical trial of the effect of yoghurt on the human salivary microflora. Arch Oral Biol.46: 705-712.

Petti S, Tarsitani G and Simonetti D'Arca A. 2008. Antibacterial activity of yoghurt against viridans streptococci *in vitro*. Arch Oral Biol. 53(10): 985-990.

Peuhkuri K, Lähteenmäki T, Sievi E, Saxelin M, Vapaatalo H and Korpela R. 1996. Antioxidative properties of *Lactobacillus* GG measured as prostacyclin and nitric oxide production in endothelial cell culture. Nutr Today. (Suppl.) 31: 53S-54S.

Piaia M, Antoine JM, Guardia JAM, Leplingard A and Wijnkoop IL. 2003. Assessment of the benefits of live yogurt: methods and markers for *in vivo* studies of the physiological effects of yogurt cultures. Micro Eco Health Dis. 15: 79-87.

Picot A and Lacroix C. 2004. Encapsulation of Bifidobacteria in whey protein-based microencapsules and survival in simulated gastrointestinal conditions and in yogurt. Int Dairy J. 14: 505-515.

Piddocke MP, fazio A, Vongsangnak W, Wong ML, Heldt-hansen HP, Workman C, Nielsen J and Olsson. 2011. Revealing the beneficial effect of protease supplementation to high gravity beer fermentations using -omics techniques. Microb Cell Fact. 10:27.

Pinchuk I V, Bressollier P, Verneuil B, Fenet B, Sorokulova I B, Megraud F and Urdaci M C. 2001. *In vitro* anti-*Helicobacter pylori* activity of the probiotic strain *Bacillus subtilis* 3 is due to secretion of antibiotics. Antimicrob Agents Chemother. 45:3156-3161.

Pinto MGV, Franz CMAP, Schillinger U and Holzapfel WH. 2006. *Lactobacillus* spp. with *in vitro* probiotic properties from human faeces and traditional fermented products. Intern J Fd Microbiol. 109(3):205-214.

Plessas S, Bosnea L, Alexopoulos A and Bezirtzoglou E.2012. Potential effects of probiotics in cheese and yogurt production: A review. Eng. Life Sci.12 (4): 1-9.

Pletincx M, Legein J and Vandenplas Y.1995. Fungemia with *Saccharomyces boulardii* in a 1 year-old girl with protracted diarrhea. J Pediatr Gastroenterol Nutr. 21:113-115.

Plummer S, Weaver MA, Harris JC, Dee P and Hunter J.2004. Clostridium difficile pilot study: effects of probiotic supplementation on the incidence of *C.difficile diarrhoea*. Int Microbiol. 7(1):59-62.

Pool-Zobel BL. 2005. Inulin-type fructans and reduction in colon cancer risk: Review of experimental and human data. Br J Nutr. 93: S73 S90.

Popova M, Molimard P, Courau S, Crociani J, Dufour C, Le Vacon F and Carton T. 2012. Beneficial effects of probiotics in upper respiratory tract infections and their mechanical actions to antagonize pathogens. J Appl Microbiol. 113(6):1305-1318.

Prado F C, Parada JL, Pandey A, Socco C R. 2008. Trends in non-dairy probiotic beverages. Fd Res Intern. 41(2): 111-123.

Prescott SL, Dunstan JA, Hale J, Breckler L, Lehmann H, Weston S, Richmond P. 2005. Clinical effects of probiotics are associated with increased interferon-gamma responses in very young children with atopic dermatitis. Clin Exp Allergy. 35(12):1557-1564.

Prescott SL, Wiltschut J, Taylor A, Westcott L, Jung W, Currie H and Dunstan JA. 2008. Early markers of allergic disease in a primary prevention study using probiotics. 2.5-year follow-up phase. Allergy. 63(11):1481-1490.

Pretorius IS. 2000. Tailoring wine yeast for the new millennium; novel approaches to the ancient art of wine making. Yeast.16: 675-729.

Prevention of beta-lactam-associated diarrhea by *Saccharomyces boulardii* compared with placebo. Am. J. Gastroenterol. 90:439-448.

Prieto ML, O'Sullivan L, Tan SP, McLoughlin P, Hughes H, et al. 2012. Assessment of the bacteriocinogenic potential of marine bacteria reveals lichenicid in production by seaweed-derived *Bacillus* spp. Mar Drugs. 10: 2280-2299.

Proteins in intact bacteria during drying. Appl Environ Microbiol. 61: 3592-3597.

Psani M and Kotzekidou P. 2006. Technological characteristics of yeast strains and their potential as starter adjuncts in Greek-style black olive fermentation. World J Microbiol Biotechnol. 22:1329-1336.

Psomas E, Andrighetto C, Litopoulou-Tzanetaki E, Lombardi A and Tzanetakis N. 2001. Some probiotic properties of yeast isolates from infant faeces and feta cheese. Int J Food Microbiol. 69:125-133.

Psomas EI, Fletouris DJ, Litopoulou-Tzanetaki E and Tzanetakis N. 2003.Assimilation of cholesterol by yeast strains isolated from infant feces and Feta cheese. J Dairy Sci. 86(11):3416-3422.

Pyo HY, Lee CT and Lee CY. 2005. Effect of lactic acid fermentation on enrichment of antioxidant properties and bioactive isoflavones in soybean. J Fd. 70: S215-S220.

Qian Z J, Jung W K, Kang K H, Ryu B, Kim S K, Je J Y. et al, 2012. *In vitro* antioxidant activities of the fermented marine microalga *Pavlova lutheri* (haptophyta) with the yeast *Hansenula polymorpha*. J Phycol. 48:475-482.

Quintus J, Kovar KA, Link P and Hamacher H.2005.Urinary excretion of arbutin metabolites after oral administration of bearberry leaf extracts. PlantaMed. 71(2):147-152.

Rafter J.2003. Probiotics and colon cancer. Best Practice Research Clin Gastroenterol 17:849 859.

Raghavendra P and Halami PM. 2009. Screening, selection and characterization of phytic acid degrading lactic acid bacteria from chicken intestine. Int J Fd Microbiol. 133(1- 2):129-134.

Ragione La, Casula RMG, Cutting SM and Woodward SM. 2001. *Bacillus subtilis* spores competitively exclude *Escherichia coli* 070:K80 in poultry. Vet. Microbiol. 2062:133-142.

Rajalakshmi R and Vanaja K. 1967. Chemical and biological evaluation of the effects of fermentation on the nutritive value of foods prepared from rice and grams. Br J Nutr. 21: 467-473.

Rajkowska K and Kunicka-Styczyńska A. 2010. Probiotic propereties of yeasts isolated from chicken feces and Kefirs. Polish J Microbiol. 59 (4): 257-263.

Rajkumar C, D'Souza A L, Cooke J and Bulpitt C. 2002. Probiotics in prevention of antibiotic associated diarrhea: Meta analysis. BMJ. 324:7350.

Ramasamy K, Shafawi ZM, Mani V, Wan HY and Majeed ABA. 2012. *Hypocholesterolaemic* effects of probiotics. In: Complementary Therapies for the Contemporary Healthcare. Saad M and de Medeiros (Eds.) In Tech. 163-180.

Ranadheera, C.S., Prasanna, P.H.P., Vidanarachchi, J.K.2014. Fruit juice as probiotic carriers. In FruitJuices: Types, Nutritional Composition and Health Benefits, 1st ed.; Elder, K.E., Ed. NovaScience Publishers: Hauppauge, NY, USA. 1-19.

Rao T Surya Chandra, SB Rachappa and Agrawal Renu.2007.Role of oxygen scavengers in improving the stability and viability of *Pediococcus pentosaceus*. Res J Biotechnol. 2 (1): 26-32.

Raposo M F de Jesus, de Morais R M S C and de Morais AMMB.2013. Bioactivity and Applications of Sulphated Polysaccharides from Marine Microalgae. Mar Drugs. 11(1): 233-252.

Rasic J L, Vujicic I F, Skrinjar M and Vulic M.1992. Assimilation of cholesterol by some cultures of lactic acid bacteria and *Bifidobacteria*. Biotech Lett. 14 (1): 39-44.

Rati ER, Vijayendra SVN, Varadaraj MC, Nirmala Devi S, Agrawal R, Nand K, Prasad MS.2003. Fermentation technologies for smaller communities. J Rural Technol. 1(1):28- 32.

Ratledge C.1991. Microorganisms for lipids. Acta Biotechnol.4 (5):429-438.

Ratledge MP and Wynn JP. 2002. The biochemistry and molecular biology of lipid accumulation in oleaginous microorganisms. Adv. Appl. Microbiol. 51:1-51.

Rayes N, Seehofer D, Hansen S, et al. 2002. Early enteral supply of lactobacillus and fiber versus selective bowel decontamination: a controlled trial in liver transplant recipients. Transplantation.74:123-128.

Rayes N, Seehofer D, Theruvath T, et al. 2005. Supply of pre- and probiotics reduces bacterial infection rates after liver transplantation: a randomized, double-blind trial. Am J Transplant.5:125-130.

Reale A, Di Renzo T, Rossi F, Zotta T, Iacumin L, Preziuso M and Coppola R. 2015. Tolerance of Lactobacilluscasei, *Lactobacillus paracasei* and *Lactobacillus rhamnosus* strains to stress factors encountered in food processing and in the gastro-intestinal tract. LWT - Fd Sci Technol. 60:721-728.

Reddy K Srinath, Salim Yusuf.1998. Current Perspectives. Emerging Epidemic of Cardiovascular Disease in Developing Countries. Circulation. 97: 596-601.

Reddy K. S. 1998. Rising burden of cardiovascular diseases in India. In: Sethi KK, Ed.Coronary Artery Disease in Indians-A Global Perspective. Mumbai: Cardiological Society of India. 63-72.

Reid G and Bruce AW. 2006. Probiotics to prevent urinary tract infections: the rationale and evidence. World J Urol. 24(1):28-32.

Reid G et al. 1992. Influence of three-day antimicrobial therapy and *Lactobacillus* vaginal suppositories on recurrence of urinary tract infections. Clin Ther.14 (1): 11-16.

Reid G, Bruce AW, Fraser N, Heinemann C, Owen J and Henning B.2001. Oral probiotics can resolve urogenital infections. FEMS immunol Med Microbiol.http://dx.doi.org/10.1111/j.1574-695X.2001.tb01549.x

Reid G, et al. 2001. Probiotic *Lactobacillus* dose required to restore and maintain a normal vaginal flora. FEMS Immunol Med Microbiol. 32: 37-41.

Reid G, Howard J and Gan B S. 2001. Can bacterial interference prevent infection. Trend. Microbol. 9:424-428.

Reid G, Jass J, Sebulsky M T and McCormick J K. 2003. Potential uses of probiotics in clinical practice. Clin Microbiol. Review. 16:658-672.

Reid G, McGroarty JA, Angotti R and Cook RL.1988. Lactobacillus inhibitor production against *Escherichia coli* and coaggregation ability with uropathogens. Can J Microbiol. 34:344-351.

Reid G. 2002. Probiotics for urogenital health. Nutr Clin Care. 5:3-8.

Reid G. 2010. The potential role for probiotic yogurt for people living with HIV/AIDS.Gut Microbes.1 (6):411-414.

Ren D, Li C, Qin Y, Yin R, Du S, Ye F, et al. 2014. *In vitro* evaluation of the probiotic and functional potential of *Lactobacillus* strains isolated from fermented food and human intestine. Anaerobe. 30: 1-10.

Ren D, Li C, Qin Y, Yin R, Li X, Tian M, Du S, Guo H, Liu C, Zhu N, SunD, Li Y and Jin N. 2012. Inhibition of *Staphylococcus aureus* adherence to Caco-2 cells by *Lactobacilli* and cell surface properties that influence attachment. Anaerobe.18:508-515.

Renu Agrawal and Shylaja Dharmesh. 2011. An antishigella protein from *Pediococcus pentosaceous* MTCC 5151. Turk J Biol. 36: 177-185.

Renu Agrawal, Rati Rao ER, Vijayendra SVN, Varadaraj MC, Prasad MS and Krishna Nand. 2000. Flavour profile of idli batter prepared for defined microbial starter cultures. World J Microbiol Biotechnol.16: 687-690.

Renu Agrawal, Vanaja G, Villetchka Gotcheva and Angel Angelov. 2010. Differences in biochemical and electrophoretic properties in native *Lactobacillus plantarum* and probiotic culture strain *Lactobacillus plantarum* cfr on adaptation to GIT conditions with functional properties. Research Journal of Biotechnology. 5 (2): 67-73.

Richelsen B, Kristensen K and Pedersen SB.1996. Long-term (6 months) effect of a new fermented milk product on the level of plasma lipoproteins – a placebo-controlled and double blind study. Eur JClin Nutr. 50: 811-815.

Rincon Delgadillo PA. *et al.* 2012. Implementation of a chemo-epitaxy flow for directed self-assembly on 300 mm wafer processing equipment. J Micro/Nanolithography, MEMS, and MOEMS. 031302-1:031302-5.

Ritter J M. 2011. Dual blockade of the renin-angiotensin system with angiotensin converting enzyme (ACE) inhibitors and angiotensin receptor blockers (ARBs). Br J Clin Pharmacol. 71(3):313-315.

Rivera-Espinoza Y, Gallardo-NavarroY. 2010. Non-dairy probiotic products. Fd Microbiol. 27(1):1-11.

Rodriguez E, Gonzalis B, Gaya P, Neunez M and Medina M.2000. Diversity of bacteriocins produced by lactic acid bacteria isolated from raw milk. Intl Dairy J.10:7-15.

Rolfe R D. 2000. The role of probiotic cultures in the control of gastrointestinal health. J Nutri. 396s-402s.

Rook GA, Brunet LR. 2005. Microbes, immunoregulation, and the gut.Gut. 54(3):317-320.

Rorick MH and Scrimshaw NS.1979. Comparative tolerance of elderly from differing ethnic backgrounds to lactose-containing and lactose-free dairy drinks: a double-blind study. J Gerontol. 34:191-196.

Rosenberg M, Gutnick D and Rosenberg E.1980. Adherence of bacteria to hydrocarbons: a simple method for measuring cell-surface hydrophobicity. FEMS Microbiol Lett.9:29-33.

Rosenfeldt V, Benfeldt E, Nielsen S, Michaelsen KF, Jeppesen DL,Valerius NH and Paerregaard A.2003. Effect of probiotic *Lactobacillus strains* in children with atopic dermatitis. J Allergy Clin Immunol.111:389-395.

Ross R P, Desmond C, Fitzgerald G F and Stanton C. 2005. Overcoming the technological hurdles in the development of probiotic foods. J. Appl Microbiol. 98:1410-1417.

Ross R P, Stanton C, Hill C, Fitzgerald G F and Coffey A. 2000. Novel cultures for cheese improvement. Trends Fd Sci Technol. 11:96-104.
Roy D and Ward P. 1990. Evaluation of rapid methods for differentiation of *Bifidobacterium* species. J Appl Bacteriol. 69:739-749.
Saarela M, Mogensen G, Fonden R, Matto J and Sandholm T. 2000. Probiotic bacteria: safety, functional and technological properties. J Biotechnol. 84: 197-215.
Saarela M, Virkajärvi I, Alakomi HL, Sigvart-Mattila P and Mättö J. 2006. Stability and functionality of freeze-dried probiotic *Bifidobacterium* cells during storage in juice and milk. Int Dairy J. 16:1477-1482.
Saavedra JM, Bauman NA, Oung I, Permen JA and Yolken RH.1994. Feeding of *Bifidobacterium bifidum* and *Streptococcus thermophilus* to infants in hospital. Lancet. 344:1046-1049.
Sabbi T, De Angelis P, Colistro F, Dall'Oglio L, di Abriola GF, Castro M. 2005. Efficacy of noninvasive tests in the diagnosis of *Helicobacter pylori* infection in pediatric patients. Arch Pediatr Adolesc Med.159 (3):238-241.
Saberi S, Cliff M A and van Vuuren H J J. 2012. Impact of mixed S. cerevisiae strains on the production of volatiles and estimated sensory profiles of Chardonnay wines. Fd Res Int. 48:725-735.
Sah B N, Vasiljevic T, McKechnie S, Donkor O N. 2014. Effect of probiotics on antioxidant and antimutagenic activities of crude peptide extract from yogurt. Fd Chem. 156: 264-270.
Salminen S and Deighton M. 1992. Lactic acid bacteria in the gut in normal and disordered states. Dig Dis.10:227-238.
Salminen S and Tanaka R. 1995. Annual review on cultured milks and probiotics. IDF Nutri Newslett. 4:47-50.
Salminen S, von Wright A, Morelli L, et al.1998. Demonstration of safety of probiotics–a review. Int J Fd Microbiol. 44:93-106.
Salminen S. 1990. The role of intestinalmicrobiota in preserving intestinal integrity and health with special reference to lactic acid bacteria. Ann Med. 22: 42.
Salminen S.2001. Human studies on probiotics: Aspects of scientific documentation. Scand J Nutri. 45:8-12.
SalminenS, Lee YK and Playne M. 2003. Successful Probiotic *Lactobacilli*: Human Studies on Probiotic Efficacy. In: Handbook of Functional Dairy Products, Shortt, C. and J.O. AoBrien (Eds.) CRC Press, USA.
Saloff-Coste CJ.1995. Diarrhea and fermented milks. Danone World Newsletter 8:1-8.
Sanders M E. 1998. Development of Consumer Probiotics for the U.S. Market. Brit J Nutr. 80(Suppl.2): S213-218.
Sanders ME and Klaenhammer TR.2001.The scientific basis of *Lactobacillus acidophilus* NCFM functionality as a probiotic. J Dairy Sci.84 (2):319-31.
Sanders ME. 1994. How healthful is yogurt? Healthline.13:8.
Sanders ME. 2008. Use of probiotics and yogurts in maintenance of health. J Clin Gastroenterol. 42 Suppl 2:S71-S74.
Sanders ME.1995. Lactic acid bacteria and human health. In: Fuller R, Heidt P, Rusch V and van derWaaij D (Eds.) Probiotics: Prospects of Use in Opportunistic Infections. Institute for Microbiology and Biochemistry, Herborn, Germany.126-140.
Sanders ME. 2000. Considerations for use of probiotic bacteria to modulate human health. J Nutr.130 (2S Suppl): 384S-390S.
Sandine WE.1996. Commercial Production of Dairy Starter Cultures. In: Dairy Starter Cultures, Cogan, T.M. and J.P. Accolas (Eds.). Wiley-VCH, New York. 191-206.
Sanni AI and Lonner C.1993. Identification of yeasts isolated from Nigerian traditional alcoholic beverages. Fd Microbiol. 10: 517-523.

Santivarangkna C, Kulozik U and Foerst P. 2007. Alternative Drying Processes for the Industrial Preservation of Lactic Acid Starter Cultures. Biotechnol Prog. 23(2): 302-315.

Sarra PG, Morelli L and Bottazzi V. 1992. The lactic acid microflora of fowl. In this lactic acid bacteria. The lactic acid bacteria in Health and Disease Ed. Wood BJB. London, New York: Elsevier Applied Science. 1: 3-21.

Satokari RM, Vaughan EE, Smidt H, Saarela M, Matto J and Willem M de Vos. 2003. Molecular approaches for the detection and identification of *Bifidobacteria* and *Lactobacilli* in the human gastrointestinal tract. Syst Appl Microbiol. 26: 572-584.

Sauerwein H, Schmitz S, Hiss S. 2007. Effects of a dietary application of a yeast cell wall extract on innate and acquired immunity on oxidative status and growth performance in weanling piglets and on the ileal epithelium in fattened pigs. J Anim Physiol Anim Nutr. (Berl.) 91: 369-380.

Saurabh (Rob) Aggarwal, Kumar S and Topaloglu J. 2012. Novel Health Strategies. Probiotics significantly reduce mortality in preterm newborns with Necrotisin genterocolitis: results of large network meta-analysis. www. Novelhealth strategies.com

Savaiano DA. 2011. Lactose Intolerance: An Unnecessary Risk for Low Bone Density. In: Clemens et al. (Hg): Milk and Milk Products in Human Nutrition. Nestlé Nutrition Institute Workshop, Pediatric Program. 67: 161-171.

Savijoki K, Ingmer H and Varmanen P. 2006. Proteolytic systems of lactic acid bacteria. Appl Microbiol Biotechnol. 71: 394-406.

Saxelin M, Lassig A, Karjalainen H, Tynkkynen S, Surakka A, Vapaatalo H, Järvenpää S, Korpela R, Mutanen M and Hatakka K.2010. Persistence of probiotic strains in the gastrointestinal tract when administered as capsules, yoghurt, or cheese.Int J Fd Microbiol.15, 144(2): 293-300.

Sazawal S, Hiremath G, Dhingra U, Malik P, Deb S, Black RE. 2006. Efficacy of probiotics in prevention of acute diarrhoea: a meta-analysis of masked, randomised, placebo-controlled trials. Lancet Infect Dis. (6): 374-382.

Scarpellini E, Cazzato A, Lauritano C, Gabrielli M, Lupascu A, Gerardino L, Abenavoli L, Petruzzellis C, Gasbarrini G, Gasbarrini A.2008. Probiotics: which and when? Dig Dis.6 (2):175-182.

Schaafsma G. 1993. Lactose intolerance and consumption of cultured dairy products – a review. IDF Nutri Newslett. 2:15-16.

Scheinbach S.1998. Probiotics: Functionality and commercial status. Biotech. Adv. 16(3): 581-608.

Schiffrin E, Brassart D, Servin AL, Rochat F and DonnetHughes A.1997. Immune modulation of blood leukocytes in humans by lactic acid bacteria: criteria for strain selection. Am J Clin Nutr. 66: 15-20.

Schiffrin EJ, Rochat F, Link-Amster H, Aeschlimann JM and Donnet-Hughes A. 1995. Immunomodulation of human blood cells following the ingestion of lactic acid bacteria. J Dairy Sci.8:491-497.

Schillinger U, Guigas C and Holzapfel WH. 2005. *In vitro* adherence andother properties of Lactobacilli used in probiotic yogurt-like products.Int Dairy J. 15: 1289-1297.

Schlimme E and Meisel H.1995. Bioactive peptides derived from milk proteins. Structural, physiological and analytical aspects. Die Nahrung. 39: 1-20.

Schnurer J and Jonsson A. 2011. Pichia Anomala J121: a 30-year over night near success biopreservation story.Antonie Van Leeuwenhoek. 99: 5-12.

Scholmerich J. 2007. Treatment of inflammatory bowel disease. Schweiz. Rundsch Med Prax. 96:337.

Schrezenmeir J,de Vrese M.2001. Probiotics, prebiotics and synbiotics–approaching a definition. Am J Clin Nutr. 73:361-364.

Schultz M. and Sartor RB. 2000. Probiotics and inflammatory bowel diseases. Am J Gastroenterol. 95: 19S-21S.

Scott M Grundy, Gary JBalady, Michael H Criqui, Gerald Fletcher, Philip Greenland, Loren F Hiratzka, Nancy Houston-Miller, Penny Kris-Etherton, Harlan M Krumholz, John LaRosa, Ira S Ockene, Thomas A Pearson, James Reed, Reginald Washington and Smith Jr. 1998. Primary prevention of coronary heart disease: guidance from Framingham: a statement for healthcare professionals from the AHA Task Force on Risk Reduction. American Heart Association.Circulation. 97: 1876-1887

Senz M, Lengerich BV, Bader J and Stahl U. 2015. Control of cell morphology of probiotic *Lactobacillus acidophilus* for enhanced cell stability during industrial processing. Int J Fd Microbiol. 192(1): 34-42.

Serban DE. 2014. Gastrointestinal cancers: influence of gut microbiota, probiotics and prebiotics. Cancer Lett. 10; 345(2):258-270.

Sergio Ammendola, 2001. Characterization of *Bacillus* Species used for Oral Bacteriotherapy and Bacterioprophylaxis of Gastrointestinal Disorders. Appl Environ Microbiol. 66(12): 5241-5247.

Serraino M R, Thompson L U, Savoie L and Parent G. 1985. Effect of phytic acid. On the *in vitro* rate of digestibility of rape seed protein and amino acid. J Fd Sci. 50: 1689-1692.

Severson DK.1998. Lactic acid fermentations. In: Nagodawithana TW and Reed G. Eds. Nutritional Requirements of Commercially Important Microorganisms. Milwaukee: Esteekay Assoc. 258-297.

Shah N and Prajapati JB. 2014. Effect of carbon dioxide on sensory attributes, physico chemical parameters and viability of Probiotic *L. helveticus* MTCC 5463 in fermented milk. J Fd Sci Technol. 51(12): 3886-3893.

Shah NP. 2000. Probiotic bacteria: selective enumeration and survival in dairy foods. J Dairy Sci. 83: 894-907.

Shah NP. 2007. Functional cultures and health benefits. Int Dairy J. 17:1262-1277.

Shahani KM and Chandan RC. 1979. Nutritional and healthful aspects of cultured and culture-containing dairy foods. J Dairy Sci. 62:1685-1694.

Sharma P, Tomar SK, Goswami P, Sangwan V, Singh R. 2014. Antibiotic resistance among commercially available probiotics. Fd Res Intern. 57:176-195.

Sherman P M, Johnson-Henry K C, Yeung H P, Ngo PSC, Goulet J and Tompkins T A. 2005. Probiotics reduce enterohemorrhagic *Escherichia coli* O 157: H7 and enteropathogenic *E. Coli* O127: H6 induced changes in polarized T84 epithelial cell monolayers by reducing bacterial adhesion and cytoskeletal rearrangements. Infect. Immun. 2005, 73(8): 5183.

Sheth, Anish A, Garcia-Tsao and Guadalupe 2008. Probiotics and Liver Disease J Clin Gastroenterol: 42: S80-S84.

Shewry PR. 2007. Improving the protein content and composition of cereal grains. J Cereal Sci. 46: 239-250.

Shobharani P, Ramesh B and Renu Agrawal. 2006. Strain improvement by mutagenesis and optimum conditions for culture parameters by response surface methodology for lactose tolerance in a novel native culture isolate *Leuconostoc mesenteroides* sub sp. Res J Biotechnol. 1(2): 5-11.

Shobharani P and Renu Agrawal. 2010. Interception of quorum sensing signal molecule by furanone to enhance shelflife of fermented milk. Fd Cont. 21 (1): 61-69.

Shobharani P and Renu Agrawal. 2007. Therapeutic importance of volatile compounds produced by *Leuconostoc paramesenteroides*. Turk J Biol. 31:35-40.

Shobharani P and Renu Agrawal. 2008. Effect on cellular membrane fatty acids in the stressed cells of *Leuconostoc mesenteroides* sub sp. Dextranicum. A native probiotic lactic acid bacterium. Fd Biotechnol. 22: 47-63.

Shobharani P and Renu Agrawal 2010. Enhancement of cell stability and viability of probiotic Leuconostoc mesenteroides MTCC 5209 on freeze drying to be used in food formulation. Intern J Fd Sci Nutr. 60 (56): 70-83.

Shobharani P and Renu Agrawal 2011. Isolation and characterization of lactic acid bacteria from cheddar cheese as a potent probiotic strain. Ind J Microbiol. 51 (3): 251-258.

Shoria A B and Ahmad S B. 2015. Survival of *Bifidobacterium bifidum* in cow- and camel-milk yogurts enriched with Cinnamomum verum and *Allium sativum*. J Ass Arab Univ Basic and Appl Sci.18:7-11.

Siddiqui MS et al, 2012. Advancing secondary metabolite biosynthesis in yeast with synthetic biology tools. FEMS Yeast Res. 12(2):144-170.

Sidhu H, Holmes R P, Allison M J and Peck A B. 1999. Direct Quantification of the Enteric Bacterium Oxalobacter formigenes in Human Fecal Samples by Quantitative Competitive-Template PCR. J Clin Microbiol. 37(5): 1503-1509.

Sidhu H, Hoppe B, Hesse A, Tenbrock K, Brömme S, Rietschel E, Peck AB.1998.Absence of Oxalobacter formigenes in cystic fibrosis patients: a risk factor for hyperoxaluria. Lancet. 352(9133):1026-1029.

Sidira M, Kandylis P, Kanellaki M and Kourkoutas Y.2015. Effect of immobilized *Lactobacillus casei* on the evolution of flavor compounds in probiotic dry-fermented sausages during ripening. Meat Sci. 100:41-51.

Sieber R, Stransky M, de Vrese M. 1997. Laktoseintoleranz und Verzehr von Milch und Milch produkten. (Lactose intolerance and consumption of milk and milk products.) Zeitschrift für Ernährungswissenschaft.36:375-93 (in German).

Simark-Mattsson C, Emilson CG, Hakansson EG, Jacobsson C, Roos K and Holm S. 2007. *Lactobacillus*-mediated interference of mutans *Streptococci* in caries-free vs. caries-active subjects. Eur J Oral Sci. 115:308-314.

Simatos D, Blond G, Le Meste M and Morice M. 1994. Conservation des bactéries lactiques par congelation et lyophilisation. In: Bacteries lactiques. Lorica, Uriage. France.169-207.

Simone De C, Rosati E, Moretti S, Bianchi SB, Vesely R and Jirillo E. 1991. Probiotics and stimulation of the immune response. Eur J Clin Nutri. 45 (2 Suppl.): 32-34.

Simonsson A. 1995. Fodermedel till svin Uppsala: Sveriges Lantbruksuniversitet, SLU Info reporter.

Sindhu SC and Khetarpaul N.2003. Fermentation with one step single and sequential cultures of yeast and lactobacilli. Effect on antinutrients and digestibies (*in Vitro*) of starch and protein in an indigenously develop food mixture. Plant Fd Hum Nutr. 58:1-10.

Sindhu SC, Khetarpaul N. 2003. Effect of feeding probiotic fermented indigenous food mixture on serum cholesterol levels in mice. Nutr. Res. 23:1071-1080.

Singh K, Kallali B, Kumar A and Thaker V. 2011. Probiotics: A review.Asian Pacific J Trop Biomed. 287-290.

Singh SP and P Sen. 2003. Coronary Heart Disease: The Changing Scenario.Ind J Prev Soc Med. 34: 1-2.

Siriwardena AK, Mason JM, Balachandra S, Bagul A, Galloway S, Formela L,et al. 2007. Randomised, double blind, placebo controlled trial of intravenous antioxidant (n-acetyl cysteine, selenium, vitamin C) therapy in severe acute pancreatitis. Gut. 56(10): 1439-1444.

Siuta-Cruce P and Goulet J. 2001. Improving probiotic survival rates. Fd Technol 55: 36-42.

Sjovall J.1959. Dietary glycine and taurine on bile acid conjugation in man: bile acids and steroids. Proc Soc ExpBiol Med. 100:676-678.

Smit HH, Engering A, van der Kleij D, de Jong EC, Schipper K, van Capel TMM, Zaat BAJ, Yazdanbakhsh M, Wierenga EA, van Kooyk Y, Kapsenberg ML.2005. Selective probiotic bacteria induce IL-10-producing regulatory T cells *in vitro* by modulating dendritic cell

function through dendritic cell-specific intercellular adhesion molecule 3-grabbing nonintegrin. J Allergy Clin Immunol.115 (6):1260-1267.
Soghra K, Hosseini M, Hamideh; Mohammad T, Mohammad RN, Abbas AIF. 2012. Probiotics as an Alternative Strategy for Prevention and Treatment of Human Diseases: A Review. Source: Inflammation & Allergy-Drug Targets (Formerly Current Drug Targets Inflammation & Allergy). 11(2) 79-89.
Sonia Michail. 2009. The role of Probiotics in allergic diseases. Allergy Asthma Clin Immunol.5 (1): 5.
Sorek R, Kunin V, Hugenholtz P. 2008. CRISPR-a widespread system that provides acquired resistance against phages in bacteria and archaea. Nat Rev Microbiol.6:181-186.
Sørensen L M, Gori K, Petersen MA, Jespersen L and Arneborg N. 2011. Flavour compound production by Yarrowia lipolytica, *Saccharomyces cerevisiae* and *Debaryomyces hansenii* in a cheese-surface model. Int Dairy J. 21:970-978.
Sourabh A, Kanwar S S and Sharma O P.2011. Screening of indigenous yeast isolates obtained from traditional fermented foods of western Himalayas for probiotic attributes. J Yeast Fung Res.2(8): 117-126.
Stamatova I and Meurman JH. 2009. Probiotics: health benefits in the mouth. Am J Dent. 22(6):329-38.
Stamer JR, Stoyla BO, Dunkel BA.1971. Growth rates and fermentation patterns of lactic acid bacteria associated with the sauerkraut fermentation. J Milk Fd Technol. 34(11):521- 525.
Stanton C, Desmond C, Coakley M, Collins JK, Fitzgerald G and Ross RP. 2003a. Challenges facing development of probiotic containing functional foods. In: Handbook of Functional Fermented Foods. Ch. 11 Ed. Farnworth, E.R. Boca Raton, FL: CRC Press.
Stanton C, Desmond C, Fitzgerald G and Ross RP. 2003b. Probiotic health benefits - reality or myth? Aust J Dairy Technol. 58:107-113.
Stanton C, Gardiner G, Meehan H, Collins K, Fitzgeralg G, Lynch PB and Ross RP. 2001. Market potential for probiotics.Am J Clin Nutr. 73: 476s-483s.
Stecksén-Blicks C, Sjöström I and Twetman S. 2009. Effect of long-term consumption of milk supplemented with probiotic lactobacilli and fluoride on dental caries and general health in preschool children: A cluster-randomized study. Caries Res.43:374-381.
Steed H, Macfarlane GT and Macfarlane S. 2008. Prebiotics, synbiotics and inflammatory bowel disease. Mol Nutr Fd Res. 52: 898-905.
Steinkraus KH.1996. Handbook of Indigenous Fermented Foods. Marcel Dekker, Inc.
Stiles ME and Holzapfel WH.1997. Lactic acid bacteria of foods and their current taxonomy. Intern JFd Microbiol. 36: 1-29.
Suarez FL, Savaiano DA, Levitt MD. 1995. A comparison of symptoms after the consumption of milk or lactose-hydrolyzed milk by people with self-reported severe lactose intolerance. N Engl J Med.333:1-4.
Sudha N, Shobharani P and Renu Agrawal. 2006. Studies on the stability and viability of a local probiotic isolate Pediococcus pentosaceous (MTCC 5151) under induced gastrointestinal tract conditions.J Fd Sci Technol. 43 (6): 677-678.
Sugawara G, Nagino M, Nishio H, et al. 2006. Perioperative synbiotic treatment to prevent postoperative infectious complications in biliary cancer surgery: a randomized controlled trial. Ann Surg. 244:706-714.
Sultana K, Godward G, Reynolds N, Arumugaswamy R, Peiris P, Kailasapathy K. 2000. Encapsulation of probiotic bacteria with alginate-starch and evaluation of survival in simulated gastrointestinal conditions and in yoghurt.Int J Food Microbiol. 5, 62(1-2):47 55.
Surawic C M. 2008. Role of probiotics in antibiotic-associated diarrhea, Clostridiumdifficile associated diarrhea, and recurrent Clostridium difficile-associated diarrhea. 64-70.

Surya Chandra Rao, Rachappa SB, and Renu Agrawal. 2007. Role of oxygen scavengers in improving the stability and viability of probiotic lactic acid bacteria. Res J Biotechnol. 2 (1): 26-32.

Suto H, Matsuda H, Mitsuishi K, Hira K, Uchida T, Unno T, et al, 1999. NC/Nga mice: a mouse model for atopic dermatitis. Int Arch Allergy Immunol. 120 Suppl 1:70-75.

Svanberg U. 1995. Lactic acid fermented foods for feeding infants. In: Steinkraus KH, editor. Hand book of indigenous fermented foods. New York: Marcel Dekker. 310-347.

Swaneck G E and Fishman J. 1988. Covalent binding of the endogenousestrogen 16 alpha hydroxyestrone to estradiol receptor in human breastcancer cells: characterization and intranuclear localization. Proc Natl Acad Sci.U.S.A. 85: 7831-7835.

Swidan N. 2009. Factors Affecting the Growth and Survival of Probiotic in Milk. Thesis. Cardiff School of Health Sciences. University of Wales Institute. Cardiff.

Szajewska H and Mrukowicz J. 2005. Meta-analysis: non-pathogenic yeast *Saccharomyces boulardii* in the prevention of antibiotic-associated diarrhea. Alim Pharmacol Therapeut. 22(5): 365-494.

Szajewska H, Ruszczyñski M and Radzikowski A. 2006. Probiotics in the prevention of antibiotic-associated diarrhea in children: a meta-analysis of randomized controlled trials. 367-372.

Szymañski H, Pejcz J, Jawieñ M, Chmielarczyk A, Strus M and Heczko PB.2006. Treatment of acute infectious diarrhoea in infants and children with a mixture of three *Lactobacillus rhamnosus* strains: a randomized, double-blind, placebo-controlled trial. Aliment Pharmacol Ther. 23(2):247-253.

Tahri K, Crociani J, Ballongue J and Schneider F. 1995. Effects of three strains of bifidobacteria on cholesterol. Lett. Appl. Microbiol.21:149-151.

Tahri K, Grill JP and Schneider F. 1996. Bifidobacteria strain behavior toward cholesterol: Coprecipitation with bile salts and assimilation.Curr Microbiol. 33: 187-193.

Taipale T, Pienihäkkinen K, Alanen P, Jokela J and Söderling E. 2013. Administration of *Bifidobacterium animalis* sub sp. lactis BB-12 in early childhood: A post-trial effect on caries occurrence at four years of age. Caries Res. 47: 364-372.

Talwalkar A and Kailasapathy K. 2004. A review of oxygen toxicity in probiotic yogurts: Influence on the survival of probiotic bacteria and protective techniques. Compr Rev Fd Sci Fd Safety. 3:117-124.

Tamang JP. 2007. Fermented foods for human life. In microbes for human life. Eds. AK Chauhan, A verma and H Kharakwal. New Delhi, India. I.K. International Publishing House Pvt. Ltd. 73-87.

Tamang JP. 2010. Himalayan fermented foods: Microbiology, nutrition and ethnic values. New York: Taylor and Francis Group.

Tamang PJ, and Fleet GH 2009. Yeasts diversity in fermented foods and beverages pp.169-198 in Satyanarayana T., editor; and Kunze G., editor., eds. Yeast biotechnology: diversity and applications. Springer, Berlin, Heidelberg.

Tamime A Y. 2002. Fermented milks. A historical food with modern applications. Eur J clin Nut. 56: S2-S15.

Tamime A, Grady B O and Gibson G R. 2007. Chapter 1.Microbiota of human gut. Book: Probiotic Dairy Products. Blackwell Publishing Ltd. DOI, 10.1002/9780470995785.

Tamime AY.1981. Microbiology of starter cultures. In: Dairy Microbiology. 2. Elsevier Appl Sci. New York, USA.113-156.

Tammam JD, Williams AG, Noble J and Lloyd D. 2000. Amino acid fermentation in non starter *Lactobacillus* spp. isolated from Cheddar cheese. Lett Appl Microbiol. 30: 370- 374.

Tannock GW, Dashkevicz MP and Feighner SD.1989. *Lactobacilli* and bile salt hydrolase in the murine intestinal tract. Appl Environ Microbiol. 55: 1848-1851.

Taranto MP, Medici M, Perdigon G, Ruiz Holgado AP, Valdez GF. 1998. Evidence for hypocholesterolemic effect of *Lactobacillus reuteri* in hypercholesterolemic mice. J Dairy Sci. 81(9):2336-2340.

Taranto MP, Medici M, Perdigon G, Ruiz Holgado AP and Valdez GF. 1998. Evidence for Hypocholesterolemic effect of *Lactobacillus reuteri* in Hypercholesterolemic Mice. J Dairy Sci. 81 (9): 2336-2340.

Tavan E, Cayuela C, Anroine JM, Trugnan G, Chaugier C and Cassand P.2002. Effects of diary products on heterocyclic aromatic amine-induced rat colon carcinogenesis. Carcinogenesis. 23: 477-483.

Taylor A, Dunstan J and Prescott S. 2007. Probiotic supplementation for the first 6 months of life fails to reduce the risk of atopic dermatitis and increases the risk of allergen sensitization in high-risk children: a randomized controlled trial. J Allergy Clin Immunol.119:184-91.

Taylor GR and Williams CM. 1998. Effects of probiotics and prebiotics on blood lipids. Br J Nutr. 80: S225-230.

The Good Scent Company (TGSC) 1989. Food additives permitted for direct addition to food for human consumption. Available at http://www.thegoodscentscompany.com/data/rw1009101.html.

Tissier H. 1905. Repartition des microbes dans l'intestin du nourisson. (Distribution of microorganisms in the newborn intestinal tract.) Ann Inst Pasteur (Paris). 9:109-123.

Todorov SD Botes M, Danova ST and Dicks LMT. 2007. Probiotic properties of *Lactococcuslactis* ssp. lactis HV219, isolated from human vaginal secretions. J App Microbiol. 103: 629-639.

Toft NJ, Winton DJ, Kelly J, Howard LA, Dekker M, te Riele H, Arends MJ, Wyllie AH, Margison GP and Clarke AR. 1999. ++Msh2 status modulates both. Proc Natl Acad Sci. USA. 96:3911-3914.

Toh ZQ, Anzela A, Tang MLK and Licciard PV. 2012. Probiotic Therapy as a Novel Approach for Allergic Disease. Front Pharmacol. 3: 171.

Tripathi MK and Giri SK. 2014. Probiotic functional foods: Survival of probiotics during processing and storage. J Funct Foods. 9:225-241.

Trois L, Cardoso EM, Miura E. 2008. Use of probiotics in HIV-infected children: a randomized double-blind controlled study. J Trop Pediatr. 54: 19-24.

Truss CO.1978. Tissue injury induced by Candida albicans, mental and neurological manifestations. J Orthomol Psychiatry.7:17-37.

Tschudy JJ and Scranton SE. 2013. Pediatrics Pre- and Postnatal Lactobacillusreuteri Supplementation decreases allergy responsiveness in infancy.132: Suppl.1.

Tuomola EM, Ouwehand AC, Salminen SJ. 1999. The effect of probiotic bacteria on the adhesion of pathogens to human intestinal mucus. FEMS Immunology and Medical Microbiology 26(2):137-142.

Tursi A, Brandimarte G, Giorgetti GM, Forti G, Modeo M E and Gigliobianco A. 2004. Med Sci Monit. Low-dose balsalazide plus a high-potency probiotic preparation is more effective than balsalazide alone or mesalazine in the treatment of acute mild-to-moderate ulcerative colitis.10 (11): PI, 126-131.

Urbancsek H, Kazar T, Mezes I and Neumann K. 2001. Results of a double-blind, randomized study to evaluate the efficacy and safety of Antibiophilus in patient's with radiation-induced diarrhoea. Eur J Gastroenterol Hepatol. 13 (4): 391-396.

Uribarri J, Oh MS and Carroll HJ.1998. D-lactic acidosis. A review of clinical presentation, biochemical features, and pathophysiologic mechanisms. Medicine 77: 73-82.

Uzogara SG, Agu LN and Uzogara EO. 1990. A review of traditional fermented foods, condiments and beverages in Nigeria: Their benefits and possible problems. Ecol Fd Nutri. 24(4): 267-288.

Van den Nieuwboer M, Klomp-Hogeterp A, Verdoorn S, Metsemakers-Brameijer L, Vriend T M, Claassen E, et al. 2015. Improving the bowel habits of elderly residents in a nursing home using probiotic fermented milk. Benef. Microbes. 17:1-8.

Van den Nieuwboer M, van de Burgwal LHM, Claassen E. 2015. A quantitative key opinion-leader analysis of innovation barriers in probiotic research and development: Valorisation and improving the tech transfer cycle. Pharma Nutri. 25 September.

Van der Aa L, Heymans H, van Aalderen W, Sillevis Smitt JH, Knol J, Ben Amor K, Goossens DA and Sprikkelman AB. 2010. Synbad Study Group. Effect of a new synbiotic mixture on atopic dermatitis in infants: A randomized-controlled trial. Clin. Exp. Allergy.40:795- 804.

Van der Veen S and Abee T. 2011. Mixed species biofilms of *Listeria monocytogenes* and *Lactobacillus plantarum* show enhanced resistance to benzalkonium chloride and peracetic acid. IntJFd Microbiol. 144: 421-431.

Vanaja G, Gotcheva V, Angelov A and Agrawal R. 2011. Formation of volatiles and fatty acids of therapeutic importance in the probiotic *Lactobacillus plantarum* LPcfr adapted to resist GIT conditions. J Fd Sci Technol. 48(1):110-113.

Vanderhoof JA. 2000. Probiotics and intestinal inflammatory disorders in infants and children. J Pediatr Gastroenterol Nutr. 30: S34-S38.

Vanitha R and Renu Agrawal. 2012. Purification of protein from probiotic *Leuconostoc mesenteroides* active against V. cholerae. Res J Biotechnol. 7 (1): 38-42.

Vankerckhoven V, Huys G, Vancanneyt M, Vael C, Klarel, Romond MB, EntenzaJ, Moreillon P, Wind R, KnowJ,Wiertz E,Pot B,Vaughn E, Kahlmeter G and Goossens H. 2008. Biosafety assessment of probiotics used for human consumption: recommendations from the EU PROSAFE project. Trends Fd Sci. Technol. 19:102-114.

Vasiljevic T and Shah NP.2007. Fermented milk: health benefits beyond probiotic effect. In: Handbook of food product manufacturing. Hui YH, Eds. Vol. 2: Hoboken N.J. JohnWiley & Sons Inc. 99-116.

Vecchi E De and L Drago. 2006. *Lactobacillus sporogenes* or *Bacillus coagulans*: misidentification or mislabelling? Intern J Prob Prebio. 1(1): 3-10.

Veckman V, Miettinen M, Matikainen S, Lande R, Giacomini E, CocciaEM, Julkunen I. 2003. Lactobacilli and streptococci induce inflammatory chemokine production in human macrophages that stimulates Th1 cell chemotaxis. J Leukoc Biol.74(3): 395- 402.

Venket Rao A, Bested AC, Beaulne TM, Katzman MA, Iorio C, Berardi JM, Logan AC. 2009.A randomized, double-blind, placebo-controlled pilot study of a probiotic in emotional symptoms of chronic fatigue syndrome. Gut Pathogens.1:6.

Vesa TH, Korpela RA and Sahi T.1996. Tolerance to small amounts of lactose in lactose maldigesters. Am J Clin Nutr. 64:197-201.

Vesa TH, Marteau PR, Briet FB, Boutron-Ruault MC and Rambaud JC.1997. Raising milk energy content retards gastric emptying of lactose in lactose-intolerant humans with little effect on lactose digestion. J Nutr.127:2316-2320.

Vesa TH, Seppo LM, Marteau PR, Sahi T, Korpela RA.1998. Role of irritable bowel syndrome in subjective lactose intolerance. Am J Clin Nutr. 67:710-715.

Vesterlund S, Paltta J, Karp M and Ouwehand AC. 2005. Adhesion of bacteria to resected human colonic tissue: quantitative analysis of bacterial adhesion and viability. Res Microbiol. 156:238-244.

Vesterlund S, Vankerckhoven V, Saxelin M, Goossens H, Salminen S and Ouwehand AC. 2007. Safety assessment of *Lactobacillus* strains: presence of putative risk factors in faecal, blood and probiotic isolates. Int J Fd Microbiol.116: 325-331.

Vidya Laxme B, A Rovetto, R Grau and Renu Agrawal. 2014. Synergistic effects of probiotic *Leuconostoc mesenteroides* and *Bacillus subtilis* in ragi (*Eleucinecorocana*) malt for antagonistic activity against Vibriocholerae and other beneficial properties. J Fd Sci Technol. 51(11): 3072-3082.

Vimala Y and Dileep P. 2006. Some aspects of probiotics. Ind. J of Microbiol. 46:1-7.

Vinderola, C.G., N. Bailo and J.A. Reinheimer. 2000. Survival of probiotic microflora in Argentinean yoghurts during refrigerated storage. Food Res. Int. 33:97-102.

Vogelsang H, Ferenci P, Gangl A. 1987. Die Laktoseintoleranz. (Lactose intolerance.) Ernährung. 11:339-43 (in German).
Voltan S, Castagliuolo I, Elli M, Longo S, Brun P, D'Inca" R, Porzionato A, Macchi V, Palu" G et al. 2007. Aggregating phenotype in *Lactobacillus crispatus* determines intestinal colonization and TLR2 and TLR4 modulation in murine colonic mucosa. Clin Vaccine Immunol. 14: 1138-1148.
Von Wright, A. 2005. Regulating the safety of probiotics- The European approach. Current Pharmaceutical Design 11 (1): 17-23.
Walker GM. 2009. Fungi | Yeasts. In: Schaechter M., Ed. Encyclopedia of microbiology. Elsevier Inc, London, United Kingdom.478-499.
Walstra P, Wouters J T M and Geurts T J. 2006. Dairy sci technol. 2nd ed.CRC Press, Taylor & Francis Group.
Wang G, Zhao Y, Tian F, Jin X, Chen H, Liu X, Zhang Q, Zhao J, Chen Y, ZhangH , Chen W.2014. Screening of adhesive lactobacilli with antagonistic activity against *Campylobacter jejuni* Food Control 44 : 49-57.
Wang H H, Manuzon M, Lehman M, Wan K, Luo H, Wittum TE, Yousef A and Bakaletz LO. 2006. Food commensal microbes as a potentially important avenue in transmitting antibiotic resistance genes. FEMS Microbiol Lett. 254:226-231.
Wang KY, Li SN, Liu CS, Perng DS, Su YC, Wu DC, Jan CM, Lai CH,Wang TN, Wang WM. 2004. Effects of ingesting *Lactobacillus* and *Bifidobacterium* containing yogurt in subjects with colonized *Helicobacter pylori*. Am J Clin Nutr. 80:165-172.
Wang YH, Jiang Y, Duan ZY, Shao WL, Li HZ. 2009. Expression and characterization of a glucosidase from *Thermoanaerobacter ethanolicus* JW200 with potential for industrial application. Biologia. 64:1053-1057.
Welman AD and Maddox IS.2003. Exopolysaccharide production in lactic acid bacteria: perspectives and challenges. Trends Biotechnol.21:269-274.
WenYL, Fua LS, Lina HK, Shena CY, Chena YJ.2014. Evaluation of the Effect of *Lactobacillus paracasei* (HF.A00232) in Children (6-13 years old) with Perennial Allergic Rhinitis: A 12-week, Double-blind, Randomized, Placebo-controlled Study.Pedia Neonatol. 55(3):181-188.
Weston S, Halbert A, Richmond P, Prescott SL. 2005. Effects of probiotics on atopic dermatitis: a randomised controlled trial. Arch Dis Child. 90 (9):892- 897.
White E and Sherlock C. 2005. The Effect of Nutritional Therapy for Yeast Infection (Candidiasis) in Cases of Chronic Fatigue Syndrome. J Orthomol Med. 20(3): 193-209.
WHO Study Group. 1985. Diabetes mellitus. Report of a WHO Study Group.World Health Organ Tech Rep Ser. 727:1-113.
WHO. 2003. Chapter 1: Global Health: today's challenges.
WHO.2009 .World Health Statistics.WHO Library Cataloguing-in-Publication Data.
Williams E, Stimpson J, Wang D, Plummer S, Garaiova I, Barker M, Corfe B. 2008. Clinical trial: a multistrain probiotic preparation significantly reduces symptoms of irritable bowel syndrome in a double-blind placebo-controlled study. Aliment Pharmacol Ther.
Williams M, Pehu E and Ragasa C. 2006. Functional foods: Opportunities and challenges for developing countries. Agricultural and Rural development Notes. 19.
Williams R B. 2006. Relative virulences of a drug-resistant and a drug-sensitive strain of *Eimeria acervulina*, a coccidium of chickens.Vet. Parasitol. 135:15-23.
Wilson-Annan J, O'Reilly LA, Crawford SA, Hausmann G, Beaumont JG, Parma LP, Chen L, Lackmann M, Lithgow T, Hinds MG, Day CL, Adams JM, Huang DC. 2003. Proapoptotic BH3-only proteins trigger membrane integration of prosurvival Bcl-w and neutralize its activity.J Cell Biol.1; 162(5):877-87.

Winton Toft NJ DJ, Kelly J, Howard LA, Dekker M , Riele H te, Arends MJ, Wyllie AH, Margison GP, AR.1999. ClarkeMsh2 status modulates both apoptosis and mutation frequency in the murine small intestine: Proc. Natl. Acad. Sci. USA. 96: 3911-3915.

Wogan GN, Hecht SS, Felton JS, Conney AH and Loeh LA. 2004. Environmental and chemical carcinogenesis seminars. Cancer Biol. 14:473-486.

Wollowski I, Rechkemmer G and Pool-Zobel BL. 2001. Protective role of probiotics and prebiotics in colon cancer. Am J Clin Nutr. 73 (2 Suppl): 451S-455S.

Wood BJB. 1997. Microbiology of Fermented Foods. London, UK: Blackie Academic and Professional.

Woodford N, Morrison D, Johnson AP, Batiman AC, Hartings JG, Elliott TS and Cookson B. 1995. Plasmid- mediated Van B glycopeptide resistance in Enterococci. Microbial Drug Resis. 1: 235-240.

Woteki CE, Weser E and Young EA.1976. Lactose malabsorption in Mexican-American children. Am J Clin Nutr. 29: 19-24.

XiãoZ and Lu RJ. 2014. Strategies for enhancing fermentative production of acetoin: A review. Biotechnol. Adv. 32(2): 492-503.

Yadav H, Jain S and Sinha PR. 2007. Antidiabetic effect of probiotic dahi containing *Lactobacillus acidophilus* and *Lactobacillus casei* in high fructose fed rats. Nutri. 23:62- 68.

Yadav H, Jain S, Rastamanesh R, Bomba A, Catanzaro R and Marotta F. 2011. Fermentation technology in the development of functional foods for human health: Where we should head. Ferment Technol.1: 1-2.

Yan F and Polk D B. 2006. Probiotics as functional food in the treatment of diarrhea. Curr Opin Clin Nutri Metab Care. 717-721.

Yang H and Zhang L. 2009. Changes in some components of soymilk during fermentation with the basidiomycete *Ganoderma lucidum*. Fd Chem. 112: 1-5.

Yang Y, Guo Y, Kan Q, Zhou XG, Zhou XY and Li Y. 2014. A meta-analysis of probiotics for preventing necrotizing enterocolitis in preterm neonates. Braz J Med Biol Res. 47(9): 804-810.

Yaw, Reiferc and Miller E. 2010. Efficacy of vaginal probiotic capsules for recurrent bacterial vaginosis: a double-blind, randomized, placebo controlled study. Am J Obstet Gynecol. 203(2):120.e1-6.

Yi-Qi Du, Tun Su, Jian-Gao Fan, Yu-Xia Lu, Ping Zheng, Xing-Hua Li, Chuan-Yong Guo, Ping Xu, Yan-Fang Gong, and Zhao-Shen Li. 2012. Adjuvant probiotics improve the eradication effect of triple therapy for *Helicobacter pylori* infection. World J Gastroenterol. 21; 18(43): 6302-6307.

Yli-Knuuttila H, Snall J, Kari K and Meurman JH. 2006. Colonization of *Lactobacillus rhamnosus* GG in the oral cavity. Oral Microbiol Immunol. 21 (2):129-131.

Yong FM and Wood BJB.1976. Microbial succession in experimental soysauce fermentation. J Fd Tech.11:526-536.

Yoon HS, Ju JH, Kim H, Lee J, Park HJ, Ji Y, Shin HK, Do M, Lee JM, Holzapfel W. 2011. *Lactobacillus rhamnosus* BFE 5264 and *Lactobacillus plantarum* NR74 promote Cholesterol Excretion through the Up-Regulation of ABCG5/8 in Caco-2 Cells Probiotics & Antimicrocro. Prot 3:194-203

Yoon J S, SohnW, Lee O Y, Lee S P, Lee K N, Jun D W, Lee H L, Yoon B C, ChoiH S, Chung WS, Seo JG. 2014. Effect of multispecies probioticson irritable bowel syndrome: A randomized, double blind, placebo-controlled trial. J Gastroenterol Hepatol. 29(1): 52-59.

Yuki N, Watanabe K, Mike A, Tagami Y, Tanaka R, Ohwaki M and Morotomi M. 1999. Survival of a probiotic *Lactobacillus casei* strain Shirota, in the gastrointestinal tract: selective isolation from faeces and identification using monoclonal antibodies. Int J Fd Microbiol. 48: 51-57.

Yukuchi H, Goto T and Okonogi S. 1992. The nutritional and physiological value of fermented milks and lactic milk drinks. Diabetes Care. 17(21): 13-17.

Zhang B, Yang X, Guo Y M, Long FY. 2011. Effects of dietary lipids and *Clostridium butyricum* on the performance and the digestive tract of broiler chickens. Arch Anim Nutr. 65: 329 339.

Zhang ZF and IH Kim. 2014. Effects of multistrain probiotics on growth performance, apparent ileal nutrient digestibility, blood characteristics, cecal microbial shedding, and excreta odor contents in broilers. Poultry Sci. 93(2): 364-370.

Zhoa G and Zhang G. 2005. Effect of protection against freezing temperature rehydration median on viability of malolactic bacteria subjected to freeze drying. J Appl Microbiol. 99: 333-338.

Ziemer CJ, Gibson GR.1998. An overview of probiotics, prebiotics and synbiotics in the functional food concept: perspectives and future strategies. Intern Dairy J. 8(5-6):473-479.

Zin LZ, Marquardt RR and Zhao X. 2000. A strain of *Enterococcus faecium* (18C23) inhibits adhesion of enterotoxigenic *Escherichia coli* K88 to porcine small intestine mucus. Appl Environm Microbiol. 66:4200-4204.